Go Home *and* Grow Tomatoes

Go Home *and* Grow Tomatoes

How I survived breast cancer

Anna Remijn Derham

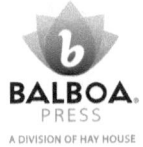

BALBOA
PRESS

A DIVISION OF HAY HOUSE

Balboa Press books may be ordered through booksellers or by contacting:

Balboa Press
A Division of Hay House
1663 Liberty Drive
Bloomington, IN 47403
www.balboapress.com.au
1-(877) 407-4847

ISBN: 978-1-4525-0832-0 (sc)
ISBN: 978-1-4525-0835-1 (e)

Printed in the United States of America

Balboa Press rev. date: 12/17/2012

CHAPTER ONE

I was lying rigid in my hospital bed, waiting for the heavy blanket of nausea to pass. Just moving my eyes caused my world to swirl around me, signalling the nausea to rise within me. My concentration was broken by the click clack sound of footsteps approaching on the polished linoleum. The clicking clacking noise was getting louder when hands of help reached towards me, pushing an empty receptacle under my bottom lip. How good did that feel to release the heaviness in my being? Well my stomach felt much better for it.

My inner voice was telling me that I would only have to lie horizontally for a short time, where I would survive this swirling of the world around me. It reminded me how lucky I was that I would not be destined to another nine months surfing the waves of morning sickness nausea that I had already survived four times some twenty or less years ago. After all now I was only recovering from the after effects of an anaesthetic. My stomach felt better but my head was swimming with questioning thoughts. Was I in the middle of a mid life crisis where everything was just happening to me? I had been anesthetised for a surgical procedure to perform a mastectomy on my left side only a few hours earlier. There was no history of breast cancer or any other cancer in my family that I knew about. There was just longevity. My Dad died just before his ninetieth birthday and my Mum died in her mid eighties. What was I doing for this to happen to me? What could I do to make it better, my life right now that is? What if I were to meditate daily starting right now? I could use creative visualisation and my imagination to help me heal. I had read how others had done it before me. I could be just like those others. I closed my eyes and pretended to meditate. It wasn't very quiet inside my head. It was like every thought in the world had lined up for a procession through my mind. I needed to clear my mind, I took a deep breath but the thoughts in my mind were still passing by. *Well that didn't work. Okay then*, I thought, *I will try concentrating on just one thought.* In fact I decided to choose a different thought from those many thoughts crowding my mind.

"Only fifty years of life had passed me by and wasn't I entitled to another fifty? What would that be like?" I asked myself. Images of the Queen and me sharing celebrations swam into my subconscious. There was an orchestra playing loud celebratory music in the background. The Queen was so close to me that I could see her. The Queen was presenting me with my 100 year birthday congratulations letter. How good was I feeling to have achieved 100 years of life? It was like watching a warm and fuzzy movie. A cacophony of voices disrupted my inner entertainment. I curiously opened my eyes to sneak a look at my surroundings.

There were other animated, talking, living bodies in the beds around me. I felt a little squeamish so I closed my eyes to regain my equilibrium. I could still listen to the chatter around me. I did however wonder what the owners' of these voices would look like. It would be a while before I could tempt fate and open my eyes again. I really didn't like feeling nauseated. My inner voice was telling me to lie still. It was like my inner voice was intent on protecting me from throwing up. Its purpose it seemed was to keep me safe by reminding me that the slightest movement would bring back the click clacking on the linoleum. I obediently lay very still not even daring to open my eyelids.

Bored with the chitter chatter of voices around me I decided to believe that simple thoughts were simple energy which would not disturb my equilibrium. If I distanced myself from my surroundings I would become the observer, who sits and would be entertained once more. In my imagination I could see in the distance that I was looking at myself lying in that hospital bed, where my golden locks bearing grey regrowth, limply splayed across my pillow. I looked so old from where I was observing. My imagination went into more play. It was like I was looking at myself way down below. I could see that I was lying very still but my hairstyles were changing. I knew in that moment that I should have kept that hairdresser's appointment earlier in the week. It suddenly occurred to me that I was lying rigid for a purpose. I was healing from an earlier procedure.

My inner voice was congratulating me. I had just taken my first significant step on my journey to rid myself of an invasive cancer. After all wasn't that the intention for my operation? I shifted in my bed to find a more comfortable position. My hand slipped across my chest where I felt that a bulge was missing; instead of two I now only had one. Images flashed through my mind of my missing bulge containing that insalubrious lump. It was sitting in a kidney dish somewhere being probed in the name of medical science. I felt that warm and fuzzy feeling again as I imagined seeing that lump of tissue that imprisoned in its centre the invasive cancer cells in their containment that which was were no longer part of me. I felt joy as I reached further into my daydream imagining that this cancer tissue sitting in the kidney dish was encased completely by a large margin of healthy tissue. My daydream had convinced me that I was clear of cancer. I even imagined that my kind surgeon dressed in his white coat was smiling with me whilst telling me that all was well in my life of health. I sensed that I felt like a vulnerable child even though my years of maturity were clearly evident. In my mind's eye this surgeon was my knight in shining armour. My creative daydream was so very real. I swear I could feel his hand in mine whilst he assured me that he got rid of all the cancer. I was convinced that I heard him tell me that no further treatment would be required. Then my daydream was interrupted.

"Mum, are you okay?" cried my boys, Sam, and Robbie in unison. I forced my eyelids to open. I could see two human forms looking down at me. I noticed that Sam my youngest son was quickly catching up in height with his older brother, or maybe he was just standing closer to the bed. I was squinting through the hospital's fluorescent back lighting which was blurring Sam's skinny frame contrasting with Robbie's more mature muscular form. I lifted my head from the pillow for a better look when I felt nausea revisit.

"Quick," I called, "I'm going to be sick." The sick bag appeared. "I'll be alright soon," I said whilst thinking, *O geez I feel so sick right now. I'll feel better this time tomorrow. Just have to give my body time to get over this; it's just the after effects of the anaesthetic.*

"I'm going to be fine," I mumbled reassuringly as my head fell back onto the pillow below. I quickly drifted back into the comfort of my foggy comatose state, knowing innately that the worst was over. My body was unmoving, relaxed perhaps, but thoughts again assaulted the momentary stillness of my mind. The more I tried to relax my mind the busier the thought traffic became. I finally settled with building on the thought that I was going to be okay. This thought took me back in time.

In my imaginings I was watching a movie on a big screen in front of me. I watched my Doctor, my General Practitioner (G.P.) who was sitting at his desk talking to me. I could see that I was seated in the chair beside his desk. He was telling me that the lump appeared to be contained and could quite possibly be a cyst. In fact, he indicated that my lymph glands appeared to be normal and unaffected. I watched myself as my facial muscles relaxed and my cheeks coloured. I remembered thinking then that I had a knowing that I was on my way to recovery from what, I was yet to discover.

Back in my hospital bed where foggy consciousness was my reality of choice, I recalled hearing that my surgery was a success. In my map of my world I perceived this information to mean that I was now clear of cancer and would need no other intervention. That was my knowledge and my reality. Imagine my shock when only a few weeks later, chemotherapy was prescribed. I remember feeling like fight, flight and freeze were kicking in instantaneously.

CHAPTER TWO

I felt so alone in my world with a small, dangerous and deadly lump that would invade every chunk of my reality. Yes I was doing overwhelm. Menopause had that effect on me too. The day I did overwhelm exquisitely well was when my youngest son Sam and I were on the road travelling to Mackay. I was filled with excitement to know that we were on our way to catch a flight from Mackay to Sydney, where Sam would compete in the High Schools National Athletics Competition. His passion and ability had led him to represent Queensland in three events, long jump, triple jump and a school relay. Sam and I were in the car on the first leg of our trip to Sydney. It was a two hour drive from home to Mackay airport.

I loved this drive through the sugar cane, growing green and thick on the flat, framed by the interesting rising hill formation, which visually changed its colours with the change in light refraction. This morning the views were awesome. The mountains were shrouded in a white mist like they had a white band around their waist, with the vegetated peaks saluting the blue skies above. However on this trip the delectable visuals were not enough to distract the awesome feelings of excitement and overwhelm that come with being the responsible menopausal parent of an achieving young athlete whose emotions in my mind were swinging between joy and fear.

"I don't know if I'm up to this," Sam grumbled.

"Like I said before Sam you have qualified, that is why you are part of the team," I said calmly. I was concentrating on the road ahead as each repeated spoken word gained intensity in my head.

"But I don't think that I deserve to be part of the team," Sam almost yelled at me. My frustration gained momentum. I reactively roared at Sam,

"Look Sam now is not the time to be telling me this." *He had watched me put so much effort into making this trip happen. I had even rolled a wheelbarrow full of grog down Main Street, selling fundraising raffle tickets to anyone who dared walk by. He should appreciate my efforts and be excited with me*, I thought. I took a deep breath, and told him once more that he deserved to be part of the team. He had after all qualified fairly and was there on his merit. *How many times had he said and how many times had I calmly reassured him that he deserved to be in the team.* I could feel my patience waning. I could feel tension rising within me, intensifying with each and every perceived aggressive word uttered by Sam.

"But I shouldn't be going, I'm not up to it," He screamed. My excitement changed to anxiety a feeling that was searing my brain. It was my hormones of course my hormones running rampant. I felt my body quiver, my gut gurgle, and my head ache

"Well do you want to go home? I can turn the car around and go home. We don't have to go," I said as I had pulled over to the side of the road ready to turn the car around towards home.

Sam shook his head and lost himself in the screen of his game boy. I watched his fingers skilfully flicker across the game controls. He was entranced in another world.

How does he do that, how does he change from grumble bum to happily losing himself in playing his Gameboy? I thought.

I sat for a moment watching him when I realised that I could feel myself shaking. I rifled through the voluminous content of my bag that seemed to have doubled in size as though it were fertilised. Sam interrupted his game boy play to curiously watch me.

"I forgot to take my medication this morning," I said. I downed my forgotten HRT tablet, my lifesaver and sanity preserver. I could feel the tablet slide down my throat pushing that anxious overwhelming feeling from my body. Whether the tablet was a placebo or not, it worked very fast to relieve my anxiety every time I took one, which was every day, except when I forgot like I did that morning. We travelled on in calm silence.

Much later that same day we arrived intact at our university style accommodation in Sydney. Sam's room was small and claustrophobic with shared bathroom facilities in the male wing.

"Hey," I said, "I'll be back to collect you for tea. I think you have a team meeting after dinner. See you then."

"Okay," responded Sam.

I left Sam immersed in his electronic world and headed for my room. I climbed stairs, walked down hallways, down more stairs and through another hallway to even more stairs. This was reminiscent of a previous life when I was a carefree tourist in Europe, eager to climb stairs and steps daily to discover new experiences at every turn. Even then my sense of direction was never one of my stronger points. I had relied on my travel companions to navigate this new world for me. I had enjoyed the experience, not worrying about which direction we were going or where I needed to go to get back to the 'kombi' van that was my home for three months. Though back in the university accommodation style rabbit warren, I was really concentrating to remember landmarks like notice boards on the walls at the end of corridors. I remembered bedroom doors with scratches or missing paint. Finally the number on the door matched the number on my key. It was actually a very pleasant room with views to a rainforest garden.

The next morning I felt the humidity envelope me as it did at home. The rainforest trees provided a canopy that was encouraging black mould to grow on some of the outside walls. Looking through the window, I caught glimpses of grey sky through the umbrella of green leaves on the huge gumtrees. This pseudo tropical environment felt familiar with the heavy muggy atmosphere signalling rain.

The smell of potential rain reminded me that it was time to find my bathroom. I remembered the concierge telling me that the key to my door opened the bathroom door as well. It was a communal female bathroom with more toilets than showers. The basins were in a line along the opposite wall to the showers with personal hygiene messages all over the wall above.

There were special notes insisting that the occupiers of these amenities take extra care to avoid further spreading of infectious bacteria causing an outbreak of illness. I looked around to find anti bacterial wipes beside the toilet seats. I sighed," Wow how lucky am I to have studied my university degree through Distance Education in the safety of my own home. I remembered that my toilets were impeccably clean when I was studying. When my studies became overwhelming I would use toilet cleaning as a distraction. I knew how to clean my toilets to a sparkling clean and when they sparkled I would return to my studies with a clearer mindset.

Back at my accommodation in Sydney I carefully wiped the toilet seat and the back of the cistern. I sat down to enjoy the relief. As I contemplated the significance of these messages around my bathroom I wondered if I was a little insane. I feared getting sick whilst so far away from home. I couldn't think of anything worse than being confined to bed and missing the adventure of exploring this unfamiliar city. Even worse would be to miss watching Sam compete.

"I'm not going to allow myself to get sick. I have too much to look forward to. I'll will myself to stay well," I remember telling myself before falling asleep.

I woke early full of anticipation for the day ahead. Butterflies raced nervously around my stomach, I was so excited for Sam. I hurried to fit in a shower before breakfast. The water felt wonderful on my skin as I stood their taking longer than usual making sure that the soap was washed away and then to my horror I felt a lump that felt like a dried pea on the underside of my left breast. My brain went into overdrive as I remembered how this lump felt exactly like the breast cancer prototype that I had felt in the Victoria College's Faculty of Nursing's open day display. Many years had passed since then but I remembered clearly how it felt. I checked and rechecked and chided myself for taking HRT. I reminded myself that I had read that HRT allegedly had side effects like breast cancer, but my HRT tablets made that anxious feeling disappear. Fear gripped my being, forcing tears to well behind my eyes. My whole life passed before me. I suddenly realised that I had too much to live for.

"I want to see my three boys grow up. My youngest son Sam is only 13 years old. I need to see my sons grow up and see them experience parenting a teenager. After all isn't that justice?" I blubbered out loud in the deserted communal bathroom.

Looking in the mirror, bits of my reflected image reminded me of my mother. "I'm getting old like her," I said to the reflected image. "But I feel so young, especially when I look from the inside out." I muttered to an empty bathroom. Avoiding my reflection in shop windows and mirrors had become a pastime for me. *I would now trade and value my self image reflected back at me, and this image, would be unconditionally loved and valued*, I thought distractedly.

"I know. I will have a lumpectomy to remove this small lump. A small lumpectomy and that way I wouldn't even notice," I assured my image in the mirror. I momentarily felt like my problem was solved. I returned to my room where I decided that this time I would keep this discovery to myself. *I'm probably overreacting anyway. It's probably nothing. Just like pimples it will more than likely disappear so what is the point of telling people. Besides they would just think I was a drama queen*, I thought.

My mind filled with thoughts that seesawed between the negativity of feeling sorry for me and the positivity of feeling that I can do something about this and that I would be able to keep it a secret. Right in the moment I needed to make a deal with God.

"All right God you have scared me, I will never take an HRT tablet ever again. I didn't think that the HRT side effects should have impacted on my health so soon. When I am eighty maybe but not in my early fifties," I said out loud in the empty bathroom.

Back in my room I systematically made my bed, tucking my pyjamas under my pillow when I realised that I had a few minutes to spare. I sat on my bed all alone in my unfamiliar room, wishing a solution to arise from within me or pour from the four walls around me.

"I don't even know where the nearest doctor is, so what's the point of worrying whilst away from home? There's nothing I can do until

I get home," I said out loud. I took a deep breath and continued my repertoire,

"M ore importantly this is Sam's time to excel. He's achieved highly to make this meet. It is a time for me to validate and celebrate with my youngest son. Nothing is going to take that away from me." I took a good look at my image in the mirror, smiled, collected my bag from on top of the cabinet in my room and locked the door behind me.

I stopped in the hallway to take a deep breath. I focused and sighed loudly. I filled my lungs for the long trek to Sam's room. I walked hallways, climbed and descended stairs until I arrived at Sam's door. I banged on the door calling loudly, "Hey Sam, are you awake?" He opened the door sparkling from head to toe. "So you enjoyed the water too? Let's go and eat before your first event so you can fuel your system." The morning was balmy as we crossed the paved quadrangle dividing the dining room from the sleeping quarters.

I am not going to share my secret with Sam. I will do what I can to distract myself to pretend that everything is fine in my life. Sam has enough to think about with his focus on today's performance, I thought to myself. I hoped that he wouldn't read my mind or detect any giveaway facial expressions. I broke through my worry and concentrated on the world around me.

Part way across the paved quadrangle I jumped as I was unexpectedly splashed with water which dribbled from my ear around my neck and down the outside of my arm. I turned catching sight of a fish pond set above the pavers on the edge of the raised garden bed. The fish were skittish and splashing as they rose to the surface. They looked at us seemingly in expectation. Wiping the water from my clothes, I looked at Sam and we laughed, "Maybe they just want to come to breakfast with us."

A few paces further down the path we passed a group of young athletes in deep conversation with their coach. I looked at Sam willing him to participate in eavesdropping with me. We nodded signalling mutual conspiracy to listen in. I was taken aback as the students were actually listening to this masterful coach. They were actually hanging on his every word and these kids were teenagers. I was hoping that Sam would feel inspired by this man's words too.

"The coach looks so serious," I whispered to Sam, "and the kids are listening intently. I must ask him about this magic"

It was like the coach was reading my mind. I heard him tell his students," I am not your parents. I'm your coach." *Ah so that is why they are attentive*," I thought as we meandered on.

From the breakfast line-up for quite a choice of hot and cold foods, I spotted Sam's favourite breakfast food, fruit loops.

"I'm not hungry," he winced as I tried to fill a plate for him. "The food here is crap and I'm not eating any of it."

One day without breakfast was no longer an issue when I could possibly be having my last breakfast very soon, I thought dramatically.

I very nearly shared my discovery with the other mum, Jan at our table. This was too big to share I would keep my secret besides it may only be a cyst and then what would people think.

"I can keep a secret," I muttered in between fake coughs. After all if you can language it, it can happen.

My fear dimmed as the images around my discovery in my mind dimmed. I felt like I was pushing these greying images to the back of my mind right back to the back of my head and way behind me. Moving these fearsome greying images further away from me helped me feel more settled. I felt like I was enabled to be totally present with Sam to plan our adventures in this big city on our days off from competition

After breakfast Sam and I found the line for the forty minute bus trip to the track. It seemed to make sense that we travel with the rest of the team.

"You haven't paid for this bus ride. Your son chose not to stay with the team therefore you didn't pay the inbuilt fees," said the scary female teacher

I was now more than ever, convinced that I had made the right decision to accompany Sam on this trip. I couldn't throw him to the wolves and expect him to perform too. Besides he was only thirteen years old.

"But Sam will miss his event if we don't come with you. No one told me there was a fee," I said quietly.

"Oh all right then, if there is room then you can catch the bus with us and we will bill you for the trip," Snarled the scary female teacher.

I subserviently agreed to her conditions. The scary female teacher had stirred memories of my own school days where I was controlled through fear in my perception of my world. We were last on the bus. Sam found a vacant seat sitting towards the back. Fortunately I had a window seat nearer the front of the bus and was able to peer out of the window where I took in flashes of scenery that smacked of accommodation density, edged by narrow roads that were filled with streaming traffic. People on the street below were walking quickly through the immensity of traffic in this over large city. So many people and even more buildings, and yet I felt so alone. I scanned the lonely scenery of many balconies crammed with outdoor furniture and potted plants. There were traces of human life where some balconies were cluttered with children's bikes and play equipment. It seemed to me that views were impersonal from these tall buildings on the busy roads with heavy traffic flows. I could smell the heavily scented air, filled with exhaust fumes and black smoke emissions from larger vehicles. I imagined that these same pungent smells would meet the nostrils of this concrete jungle's inhabitants. I was building a macabre picture of this city's community to fulfil my feelings of resentment. I imagined that I yelled to these people. *Hey I might not be here soon and my kids won't have a mother. Don't any of you care? Why would you care anyway?'* My thoughts swayed from feelings of pity for these people living in this desolation to despair as I imagined what might be ahead for me. I felt alone, but glad that I alone was the keeper of this knowledge. *I have to hide my tears or my secret will be out and Sydney won't be fun anymore for Sam and me,* I thought quietly as I bathed in the drama. I needed to distract myself before my fear turned to panic. I thought about how absolutely awesome it was that Sam was competing at an elite level. I was putting him on a pedestal thinking that he had achieved so much on just his raw ability. In my map of the world I am allowed to think what I want because it is after all my reality, my perception of my world.

The dramatic turned to sadness. I reflected on how rural living apparently condemned one to miss those opportunities for much sporting development, particularly at an elite level. I believed that if Sam chose he could make something of a career in sport but I would need to be there to make the opportunities happen. I continued to think that perhaps the athletic coach we passed in the quadrangle could coach Sam, even though this coach lived in Townsville, three hours drive north from Airlie Beach where we lived. I believed that I could make this connection work for Sam. If I die then in my mind Sam would lose his opportunity. The thought brought tears to my eyes again. My sunglasses hid these tears as I swept a glance around the bus. Groups of kids were talking and laughing and others were introducing themselves and exchanging stories about the schools they attended.

I began to think about me again. I have a job that I like, a beautiful block of land with a sea view just waiting for a house to be built on it. How long had I dreamt about having a house near the sea? Tears threatened to form in my eyes again. The reality of my sunglasses slipping down my tear streaked nose jolted my senses back to the present. I surreptitiously pushed my glasses back up my nose whilst wiping the tears with a tissue held in my other hand.

My spirits lifted as I remembered that I could use the healing skills that I had learnt at the Silva mind control seminar fifteen years prior. I told myself that I didn't need to worry as I have the notes at home somewhere. I also remembered an article I had read where Ian Gawler was reported to visualise little green men rubbing away those huge protruding cancerous lumps that threatened his life. I had time to do the same. After all the bus was travelling to the road conditions and that was very slowly. The other passengers on the bus were engaged in their own conversations. No—one noticed that I closed my eyes, relaxed and visualised little green men rubbing away at my lump. I was beginning to feel like I was taking control. I decided that I would allow myself to focus on the lump when meditating, prior to going to sleep at night or whilst sitting quietly wearing sunglasses. I was determined that Sam enjoyed his time in Sydney.

At the first opportunity we travelled into Sydney by train to play tourists. The train trip was fast only stopping at stations long enough to let passengers on or off. I watched the many huge industrial sheds with signage advertising their contents flash by us as the train picked up speed. I felt like a tiny almost insignificant part of this enormous backdrop of life. My thoughts were interrupted when a huge iron form which had survived several generations of human life loomed into view.

"Look there's the Sydney Harbour Bridge," I said to Sam.

His mouth opened, his eyes widened and his face radiated in disbelief.

"Wow this is awesome," Sam said excitedly, "We have to bring Dad, Robbie and Tom to see this." His excitement was infectious, lifting my spirits sending my imagination into overdrive once more. We were tourists open to experience this new land. The scene was set. We alighted at Circular Quay anticipating the discovery of awesome new sights.

We would experience a delectable delicacy of insatiable sightseeing in this awesome city. Even the grey skies and falling rain wouldn't dampen our spirits. Sam didn't notice the weather. He was shooting photos of the Opera House with my phone, sending them to his older brother Tom. I bathed in Sam's excitement totally distracted from my earlier serious thoughts. It was like I had pushed those serious thoughts a long way a way from me.

Sam and I watched street theatre hiding from the rain under the immense railway bridge that spanned the street. Three men dressed in spiffy suits and ties deep in conversation were stopped by the street actor, who asked,

"Did you know that one in three men is gay?"

The three men in suits stopped their conversation in mid sentence. Their jaws visibly dropped. They stared at the actor in disbelief for a few seconds and then walked on, peering over their shoulders as they walked. Sam and I laughed so much we nearly cried.

The weather reminded me of Melbourne. It changed from warm to inclement, to cold, wintry and wet in the same day. Sam and I took refuge in the warmth of McDonalds. We sat on a bar stool by the window where we could view the bustle of the outside world. In this city there was a seriousness, sophistication and friendliness in the air. Passers by were dressed, in contrast to home, very formally in their suits carrying umbrellas, and others were travelling very casually with cameras in waterproof bags. There was not a pair of shorts or thongs in sight. Sam was gnawing on his double cheese burger, the first gnaw of food for two days. We watched the number of people swell as ferries pulled into dock. It was a different world from the holiday atmosphere and ambience of the Whitsundays and suddenly much colder. I liked this place filled with its distractions of new smells, different sights and exciting experiences. I didn't want this visit to finish.

CHAPTER THREE

For five days I had tried to creatively imagine the disappearance of this pea sized lump that would change my life, but it stubbornly remained. I had shut my eyes, relaxed my body and imagined that I could see the lump. I created images in my mind to will the lump to disappear. I had imagined little green men with oversized scrubbing brushes scrubbing it away. I remembered thinking that when I took a Panadol the pain would leave almost immediately so why wouldn't this uninvited little lump disappear just as swiftly with this creative visualisation that I had decided to use to heal.

"Well this lump likes me too much to go away," I told myself.

It was then that I made a Doctor's appointment.

Just as well I have a rostered day off from work this Monday or I would have had to leave it till the following Monday, I thought trying to ease my concerns.

Sitting in the Doctor's waiting room felt like I had been waiting for an eternity before the doctor called me into his room. After the examination my doctor told me that he believed that my lymph nodes were normal and that the lump could possibly be a fibroid or perhaps a cyst, but having said that, he wasn't going to tell me to go home and forget about it, especially as I had missed my mammogram earlier in the year. It was time to share my information with my missing husband, Tim. Work had taken him to a different part of the State.

"Hello Tim, it's me. Just thought that I would let you know that I have found a lump in my breast," There was silence on the other end of the phone so I continued," I believe there is nothing to worry about. The doctor led me to believe that it is possibly a fibroid, but I need to have a mammogram just to be sure," still silence on the end of phone. I think I was trying to console myself when I continued, "Don't worry though because I don't think it is anything." I stopped to breath.

"Okay," Tim asked, "Can you call me after the mammogram anyway?"

I had convinced myself that this was a cancer scare and nothing more and telling Tim the same just reinforced my belief.

One week later I was in the car travelling south towards Mackay. Once again I left enough time to get lost, even though the hospital was on the left hand side of the main road into Mackay. Well I missed the turnoff and careered a few kilometres down the road before I could turn around. I guess I was feeling a little nervous. I had only ever had one mammogram and the thought of all that cold metal squashing parts of me was not an image I fondly remembered.

"Are you ready?" were the words I heard.

The lady taking my pictures was around sixty years old. I don't remember exactly what was said. I know that we made small talk about Christmas and family, and then it was over.

"Good I can go shopping now," I said

But the staff informed me otherwise. "Not so fast, your Doctor has ordered an ultrasound. You just need to wait outside until one of the ultrasound rooms is ready for you."

"Should I be worried?" I asked.

"It's just the usual procedure to follow a mammogram with an ultra sound," The staff said.

I waited patiently for a short while and tried to read my book. I read the same page six times it seemed but the page still looked unfamiliar. Finally I was called into the darkened room where I lay on a bed surrounded by electronic equipment. I calmly watched on the screen as the ultra sound targeted the lump. It looked like a tadpole. The lump appeared to have a body near the skin's surface and a tail pointing towards my chest wall. Then another small lump was discovered. The young lady went out to get a doctor.

"What's happening," I said trying to remain calm.

"We strongly suggest that you have a fine needle biopsy. Is that okay with you?" the doctor asked.

I nodded. Words eluded me. I panicked, my heart raced and I felt really clammy. This was getting serious now. All thoughts of shopping had left my mind. The medical staff were reassuring, trying to calm me.

"You'll know the outcome by the end of the test," informed the doctor. The room was filling with technical equipment leaving me and the bed most of the room. There was still another medical assistant expected from another hospital.

"It's not the results that concern me but that needle," I bleated. I sounded like a frightened child. No one commented. The biopsy wasn't so bad because the doctor gave me a local anaesthetic and then performed the procedure. I felt the tug and stirring of the probe as it chased cells to siphon.

"We have successfully collected cells from the larger lump but unsuccessful with the smaller lump. You will need to revisit your referring doctor to collect the results," The hospital doctor said.

"Can't you tell me now?" I begged

The hospital doctor responded, "No you will need to let the pathology doctor read the test and then send the results to your G.P."

"Can't the operator of the pathology test read the results?" I asked

"I'm sure she can but she isn't allowed to," he said

"If it is serious then I'll hear sooner rather than later, is that right?" I asked.

"Yes of course. Now have a safe trip home and don't worry," the doctor said reassuringly.

I had run out of energy to be more insistent. I sat there silently trying to make sense of this bizarre situation.

The hospital doctor smiled trying desperately to console me, "go home and try not to worry. Your doctor will have the results in the next couple of days. Just go home and don't worry."

That will give me time to collect them before heading off on Thursday to spend Christmas with my family in Brisbane. I thought.

When I finally reached the car the sun was beaming down with enough warmth to cook a chook. The hours I spent in the hospital's clinic had certainly cooled me. I was sure my bone marrow was frozen. I sat in my hot car with the windows wound up, to defrost and soak in the warmth of a hot North Queensland summer's day. I decided to ring Tim while I thawed.

"I've had the tests and I will find out the results in the next couple of days."

I held the phone to my ear and listened and then responded, "Yes, I'm sure I'm going to be alright".

I'm thawed, I thought as perspiration began to form on my top lip. It wasn't long before the car's air conditioner was on high and the car was on the road pointing towards home. I was driving away from this surreal experience, telling myself not to worry just like the doctor said. It was like I couldn't help it. I worried all the way home and continued to worry at home until my dreams broke my worry.

That same night I dreamed that I was woken from a deep sleep. "Go away. Stop pushing me out of bed. It's my bed not yours," I screamed at the big black mass, which was trying to push me out of bed. It seemed to change shape at will slipping underneath my body trying desperately to cover the mattress whilst the bulk of it cascaded towards me like a tsunami wave engulfed in a squishy big black plastic balloon form, rocking and rolling whilst it tried to take over my space.

"Get away, get away I cried." Its strength was overpowering. With every molecule of my body I mustered a huge amount of energy. "Just go away I don't want you here. It's my bed not yours." I was suddenly wide awake and fully conscious when I found myself balancing horizontally on the side of the bed. I turned and lowered my body off the bed, reaching for the floor with my feet. I ran around my flat switching on every light, scouring each room for a sign of blackness. "It was only a dream," I said aloud. But it had stirred my senses. I swear that I had seen the blackness of this mass and that I had felt a tropical condensation mist leaving traces of wetness on my skin as it pushed against me. I swear that I heard the black mass's inside sloshing like an oversized water balloon rolling down a very steep hill. The moisture smelled so sour like it was full of cat urine. I was glad that I didn't have to taste it. "It's only a dream," I repeated out loud, "Ghosts or whatever it is are not real."

I bravely got back into bed. With eyes wide open. I lay tentatively quivering in bed again waiting for daylight to save me, but it was so far away. I tried hard to will myself to sleep but I didn't dare shut my eyes should this foul mass return and overcome me. I was out of bed again pacing the rooms of my rental flat.

"I am fine it is only a dream," I said out loud over and over until I felt the swirling in my gut subside somewhat. I found a safe place behind the kitchen door where I sat on my chair with feet placed flat on the ground with my back supported in an upright position by the back of the chair. I placed my hands flat on my thighs. With my head held high I closed my eyes, pushed my thoughts aside and let my body relax. I guess I started to pray,

"Please God protect me, don't let this foul black thing back into my life. I ask you God to protect me. I believe in you God, who is love and will protect me. God is the energy within us. Our Godly energy is a link to all the godly energy. No no no God is the universe in which we live, God surrounds us. No no no God is how we live our life, purely like the preachings of Buddhism, but then what are those preachings? I'll pray to them all, one of them is bound to hear me."

I no longer cared what form God took. I sat in my chair and counted backwards from 10, taking myself deeper into a place where I felt peace flow through me. This time I managed to push my thoughts from my awareness. I felt safe. I felt freedom. I liked being in this place. I stayed for a while when on my way back to the present, I felt like I had been taken on a journey where in my minds eye I experienced and understood the mystery of death. I had visualised being with my first husband Alan's body knowing that there was more to his state than just his physical form lying peacefully in his coffin. I had elicited that same feeling that I had when I perceived that I was surrounded by Alan's energy in the room, reassuring me that everything would be okay. I sat quietly for a while. I caught a glimpse of my image reflected from the mirror above the kitchen table. I said to my image staring back at me, "How could I share this experience with anyone? They would surely think I was crazy."

The next day I decided to relate my experience with the big black blob to a spiritual friend, Natasha, who I trusted not to be dismissive. In my mind Natasha says it how it is. She listened attentively to my tale. Her short red hair framing her face intensified in redness as the colour drained from her face. "That was probably an Incubus. It is a very bad spirit that torments women in their beds. Some believe that they are sexually perverted ghosts. You must tell it to go away. It will bring bad things your way," Natasha said warningly.

"You mean I have the power of choice to accept it or make it go away?" I asked.

"Yes, you can, in fact you must tell it to go away." Natasha's gaze penetrated me almost willing me to heed her warning. I believed that Natasha knew about these things. I had experienced her tarot card readings and she knew things about me that I would never tell anyone. I thought for a moment and mumbled, "Well I did tell it to go away. Wow and I did it intuitively." I was trembling inside. I began to question my new knowledge and googled this big black blob on the internet only to be inundated with pornography sites. I found that in paranormal lore, an incubus is a spirit or demon that attacks women in their sleep. Though the orthodox believe the same experience refers to sleep paralysis. I looked further and discovered many sites referring to incubus and succubus ghosts. I thought, *if spirituality is hoo ha why do the pornographers sensationalise the idea?*

"Spirituality or ghost stuff is like electricity we can't see it but we are aware of it and know it exists," I whispered.

I started to listen to stuff. Perhaps I could describe it as sensations or an inner voice, but it didn't sound like any voices I had heard. There was a sense of urgency pushing me to find out the pathology results from the massive day before. "I know nothing is wrong. I haven't received a phone call so it can't be anything serious. It's such an imposition to go to the Doctor's," I muttered to the walls of my office, "Besides the hospital doctor encouraged me to not worry. Anyway I have too much to do getting ready for Christmas with my family down south." I hadn't seen my husband Tim and my middle son Robbie for what seemed like eons. I was tempted to defer my appointment until I returned from my holiday in Brisbane at the end of January. Christmas was a time when there was so much to do with so little time to do it in.

I was ready to leave work for the doctor's with my handbag in hand when my sister Sjanie rang from the States. "Hi, how are you?" She asked in her usual cheerful voice. I loved talking to her but I had to hurry to get to my doctor's appointment.

"Sjanie I have to go I have a doctor's appointment" I said nonchalantly

"Are you okay?" Sjanie queried.

I needed to leave or I would miss the appointment time and my Doctor was solidly booked for the rest of the day. I needed to explain the urgency of the situation. Doctor's appointments were hard to come by.

"I have a lump in my breast but I'm sure its nothing. You know how it is. I just have to go see the doctor to get my results." I thought I said quite calmly.

"I'll ring you back in about an hour. Will you be back by then?" Sjanie asked

"Yes that should be fine," I replied.

My sister Sjanie and I had become close in the last decade even though many thousands of miles separated us from California to North Queensland.

I drove from Proserpine towards Airlie Beach with the same thought repeating itself inside my head, the *test results must be clear or the doctor would be ringing me. I don't need this disruption to my working day*

My only real distraction was on the other side of my windscreen, where the immense beauty of cane fields framed by undulating blue hills, reflected the blueness of the summer sky which never ceased to amaze me. The magical scenery instilled momentary confidence within me. Under the surface I was really nervous and nearly cried when I couldn't find a free carpark close to the Doctors' surgery. Finally I found a carpark. I needed two dollars for the coin machine. I only had one dollar and ninety cents. *Oh blow it,* I thought, *I'll leave my Council name tag on the dashboard. It is a council carpark.*

"Naughty, I know but it may work, if not then I will have to pay a parking fine then so be it," I rationalised.

My next conscious moment found me waiting quietly in the waiting room kidding myself that I was reading a magazine article. I held the magazine in front of my face for what seemed like an eternity before I realised it was upside down. Then it was my turn. My test results read, "The specimen consists of numerous malignant cells."

"It can't be," I mumbled.

My G.P.'s voice had a sense of urgency in total contrast to my visit with him only days before. He said, "You have malignant cells . . ." The rest I didn't hear. My mind went into overdrive. *Cancer happened to other people not to me. Just because it felt like a cancerous lump didn't mean it was one.* I thought, *if only I could escape this nightmare.*

I wanted to run through the surgery waiting room to the vast outside world where tourists were swimming in the lagoon, where the sand meets the sea just beyond the parkland outside the doctor's surgery. I focused, imagining my escape through the door into the space outside. I could sense the sun's warmth soaking into my bare arms. I swear that I could smell the freshly cooked seafood. It was after all lunch time. Outside this door was my freedom, the paradise I wanted. Outside was where the azure sea meets the white sands with palms swaying in the breeze, where I would smell the fragrant flowers, and listen to the birds sing. My freedom would be so peacefully real but it wasn't to be my immediate reality.

Tears ran down my cheeks spilling onto my clothes, distracting my thoughts momentarily. I watched these wet spinning balls splash onto my clothes. The thoughts in my mind picked up speed, transforming negatively out of control, making me cry even more. I tried to switch my mind to positive thoughts so that I could believe in a positive outcome. I distracted myself with action plans for my immediate future, for tomorrow.

"I'm going to drive to Brisbane tomorrow," I told my G.P. who was watching me very carefully.

"I can organise an appointment with a surgeon tomorrow in Mackay," he said very assertively.

"No I'm going to Brisbane to be with my family. I'll see someone down there," I said. I was filled with fear, though I pushed it away thinking only of where I wanted to be. *I want to be with my family in our family home and they are in Brisbane.*

"Well you make sure you are in hospital having an operation next week," my GP insisted.

I had declined my doctor's offer for treatment in North Queensland and it was time to leave his surgery. I was walking out of the surgery towards the outside world where the floodgates opened. I cried buckets of tears. It seemed like I was the only one on the planet. I had a twenty minute drive to pull myself together and make all the necessary arrangements with work. I despaired as my attempt at creative healing hadn't worked. I had read that it worked for others so why not me.

"I believe in using both orthodox and alternative medicines anyway," I told myself.

"Right now I feel more confident with the orthodox medical approach. If the lump is not contained and I have to have chemotherapy and lose all my hair then maybe it won't be so bad. It may grow back thicker or curly or a different colour," I mused. I knew that I possibly faced a rocky road ahead. I decided to take it day by day. It had worked in my life before. After all I studied my university degree externally juggling work and family with a husband and three young children. I remembered how those university packages full of learning kept coming in at the beginning of each semester. They always seemed so big. The only way I could cope was to take small steps to plan the semester's workflow to meet deadlines then concentrate on the part of the reading or assignment work for that day, forgetting the mountain of other material that I needed to climb before the end of each semester.

Back in my rented unit I pulled the big suitcases from their hiding place on the top shelf of our only overstuffed clothes, linen and storage cupboard. I threw in my favourite clothes, Sam's clothes, dividing and packaging those that needed to go for recycling. I spotted the brilliant red taffeta place mats with matching red candles waiting to be mounted in their accompanying crystal candlestick holders that I was saving for my new house.

I'll take those with me to brighten up the dining room table down south. I've been saving these place mats and candles for our new house up here but they may rot and melt before the house is built, or I may. I thought.

I recalled how the planning for moving houses to our block at Hideaway Bay were roller coaster rides of high pitched excitement in expectation falling to the abysmal depths of deep disappointment. We have had two removable houses in as many years fall through at the eleventh hour.

Both times we were gazumped by evil people, I thought as tears filled my eyes. I was still so angry with the dishonesty displayed by the two parties concerned. "Arrrgh, I'm glad to be leaving this place for how long I don't know, maybe for ever," I sighed out loud.

The flat was cleaned and tidied for our eldest son Tom, to continue living there. Sam and my suitcases were packed into the car ready for an early getaway the following morning. Exhausted I fell into bed.

"It will be better down in Burpengary," I said out loud. I then lay quietly inviting sleep but my mind wouldn't let it come. The night was pleasant with a cool breeze blowing through my window across my bed. When I tilted my head to the right I could see the night sky and its twinkling stars through my open window. Suddenly my left sleeve started to flutter, as though it were caught in the breeze. How could it be, my left arm was protected from the breeze, it was my right side that should have caught the breeze. Just to freak me out a little more, I swear that I felt a gentle reassuring pat on my left arm. I slowly turned away from the window to look at my left sleeve fluttering. I remember that I clearly saw a white mass. A fluffy calm white mass just like the clouds in the sky. I lay fearfully rigid in my bed not moving a muscle because I couldn't. I remembered Natasha's advice. I could make it go away. "You just have to ask it go away," she had said.

"Go away, leave me alone, you frighten me, just go away," I said out loud.

Immediately my sleeve was still, the room felt empty. My body relaxed with relief. I was immersed in the feeling of peace and stillness. This peace was immense, filling the whole room. I lay quietly. Through my stillness I felt confidence drift into my being. I knew then that I was going to be alright. I felt that a heavy weight had been lifted from me allowing me to sleep peacefully for the first time since this roller coaster ride began. I woke to the alarm ringing at four a.m. I felt energised to face the thirteen hours of driving ahead of me.

Driving past white line after white line my noisy mind displaced the peace from the previous night and early morning. I thought about my mum, she used to tell me how sinful it was to dabble in the supernatural or deal with psychics. I've done both since mum died six years ago. My Mum believed that dabbling in stuff not sanctioned by her religion would make it tougher for me to get into heaven. I suddenly realised that her intention was to protect me. Yes that's what it must be because I haven't been struck by lightening yet. Though there was the visit from the black mass that scared me. If I wasn't scared of what went bang in the night before that I certainly was now.

My mind skipped back to the previous night. If only I hadn't freaked out and told the white shape to go away. I wonder what else I would have experienced. That's so me, panic first and think later. No matter how hard I try not to panic, I panic. "Oh well", I sighed. Thinking it was self distraction time, I inhaled deeply and exhaled. I channelled my energy to concentrate on the road ahead. I felt an overwhelming feeling of peace enter my space where my body felt comfortable and my mind was quiet. It was just like that feeling I felt the night before when the white image visited me whilst lying in my bed. I don't want this peaceful feeling to go away, I told myself in the quiet of my mind. Then it was gone.

I became aware of every bump and puddle on the road. I realised that I was taking deep breaths trying to concentrate even harder on the road in front of me. I mumbled, "I'm going to be fine. I can win this." I wanted to continue focusing on the present, but I somehow lost the how. I had discovered another lump in my groin. Thoughts swept through me uncontrollably, challenging my positivism. What if the cells had metastases in other parts of my body? What was that lump that I could feel in my groin? Wasn't it exactly like the one I felt in my left breast? Why didn't my efforts of healing visualisation work for me? These thoughts of doubt burrowed into my consciousness filling every cell in my body with fear. Tears brimmed in my eyes and overflowed down my cheeks. I focussed on the road ahead concentrating. It was hard to see through my tears. Sam was sleeping peacefully in the back seat, apparently oblivious to the struggle that was beginning to brew inside me.

Thirteen hours later in the late afternoon I arrived. Tim was waiting.

"I'm going to be fine," I said, "I have a plan." The words spilled from my mouth. "What plan?" the little voice in my head whispered. I ignored this voice. I believed that the more I assured people that I was going to be alright the more reassured I would feel.

My cancer journey was beginning and I had no real idea where I was headed. I would take one step at a time. I began by ringing phone numbers for the Doctors I knew from Melbourne who helped me with Andrew. The same Doctors who provided a mix of alternative medical and orthodox medical treatments. I had sourced their numbers through the internet where I found they were now Professors providing post graduate alternative medicine coursework for Doctors at Swinburne University of Technology. Their phones were diverted to message bank and after hour's medical numbers. It was after all just days before Christmas. I was beginning to believe that the most appropriate first step was to heed my GP's advice and have the tumour removed and very quickly.

I received so much support from my extended family. My sister rang from the States almost daily. My brother Matt had spoken with me and my older brother Jake and his wife Jill were driving up from Melbourne to spend some time with me.

My immediate family indulged me with their time and they were planning to return to the hospital as soon as they were allowed to visit me after the operation. I felt so loved and confident and so grateful to be surrounded by people who genuinely cared for me and I for them. *Who wouldn't want to fight to survive with that sort of love and support?* I thought quietly.

On January 7th 2005 I was lying on a hospital bed waiting for the anaesthetic to take. The surgical nurse listened as I told her my story," I was given the choice of a mastectomy or lumpectomy followed by radiotherapy. I believed that the mastectomy would be a safer bet and that's the way I felt the surgeon encouraged me." I remember hearing the nurse say that if it were the surgeon's testes being removed then he would be thinking differently. I remember laughing and then I remember the surgeon appearing in a floral surgical head piece.

"I like your hat," I said. The surgeon smiled kindly. I remember waiting to be wheeled into surgery and then waking in the ward.

As I lay comatose in my recovery stance I decided that taking small steps would be a good way to move forward, my mind was too fuzzy to think of the end game. I would firstly concentrate on letting the anaesthetic drugs work their way out of my system. I didn't dare move at first. Even the slightest eye movement caused a visual image of the need for a kidney dish to be shoved under my chin. *This nausea wasn't going to beat me,* I thought. My first step for my plan would be to lie very still until such time that the nausea feeling left my body. I dreamt of receiving my reward. I imagined that I could feel the hot sweet tea running down the back of my throat, whilst sitting up in bed leaning against pumped up pillows which supported my back.

Breaking through the fabric of my dream I sensed a knowing that the anaesthesia drugs had messed with my head stirring the anxious feelings about my need to manage my impending lymphedema.

When I felt the nausea subside I caught the night nurse's attention.

"Excuse me but can you describe the Lymphedema exercises that I need to do?"

The night nurse shined her torch in my direction and took a deep breath, exhaled and said assertively," In this hospital we don't do exercise in the middle of the night." I must have looked a little distressed because she subsequently promised to organise for a physiotherapist to come and see me the following morning. The next morning I was able to shuffle down the hallway hooked up to my pole on wheels, which carried the drains connected to my side draining stuff through plastic tubes into drainage bottles.

Feedback from my surgeon's team of doctors implied to me that my surgery was successful. In fact my surgeon told me that with my positive attitude I had a good prognosis. In my reality I understood quite clearly that the cancer had been removed. It was probably sitting in a kidney dish somewhere waiting to be prodded, poked and tested or whatever it is they do with people's removed innards. Forever the optimist I believed that further treatment would be unnecessary even though the results of the lymph node harvest tests were not in yet. Though at times I found my faith wavering. *But what if my lymph nodes were cancer positive?* This thought caused my palms to sweat as I clenched my fists. I closed my eyes and tried hard to clear my mind and relax my body almost fighting for the quiet of peace to return. It seemed that the harder I tried to relax the more questions crowded into my mind. *What if the lymph nodes aren't clear? What if I have to have chemotherapy?* Thoughts were running rampant through my mind. I closed my eyes even tighter, willing my thoughts to stop. It was like they crashed and banged into each other. I felt like I was pushing a tall mound of rubble from my mind. It was then that I could feel my breathing slow down, my being felt whole and relaxed as I settled back against my pillow. I was focusing on my outcome that would be longevity for me. I needed to set goals to change how I lived my life. I needed to clear the congestion in my mind to allow clarity and positive thoughts into my world. I needed to change what I did in my life through the food I consumed, the thoughts I created, the emotions that I felt to set myself up for a longer life. My plan was beginning to take shape. For the first time in my life I actually craved healthy food, choosing salads and fruit from the hospital menu over the heavier more substantial meals. I believed that my search for how I would be okay was about to begin.

CHAPTER FOUR

"Hey I can recommend a really good homeopath," a dear family friend told me by phone. I figured it was worth a try I had after all expressed my desire to anyone who would listen that my intent was to discover the best way forward towards me having good health.

"Well they took my lymph nodes and they were clear. You would think that they would put them back if they were clear, "I said somewhat humorously.

"Well it is your life and you need to take control of your life," suggested my homeopath.

But I want you to heal me. Because that's why I am here, I thought.

There was a feeling of peace in the silence that filled the room. The homeopath sat behind his desk, taking notes and evaluating the information that I was giving to him. He looked so comfortable in his natural fibre clothes and sandals and I felt comfortable sitting with him. I believed in his healing knowledge and processes for healing.

I can be open and honest with this man without feeling threatened and he listens, I thought, *so I will say what I think.*

"I know how to heal myself," I said, "I learned the Silva mind control program fifteen years ago. I'm sure I learnt a meditation and creative visualisation in mind body healing."

The homeopath looked at me and said," Anna I too participated in the Silva program sixteen years ago and let me suggest that you know you can heal yourself but you just don't know how yet." He watched me quietly before continuing, "It is becoming apparent that you are leaning strongly towards choosing meditation and creative visualisation to heal," He said.

I left his rooms feeling confident that, for this part of my journey, my custom made homeopathic potion would rebalance me and supplementing with antioxidants would chase away the free radicals. I had spent nearly two hours with the homeopath who collected the information he needed to custom make a homeopathic potion. I was amazed how well that one little tablet made me feel.

The next day quite by coincidence Tim brought home a book for me to read by psychologist Shivani Goodman called *'Nine steps to reversing or preventing cancer and other diseases/learn to heal from within.'* It sounded interesting and provided hope. I flicked through the pages getting the gist of the information contained within the binding of this book. "Hey Tim, look at this," I yelled ecstatically, "I have a healing meditation process." I pointed to the page expecting him to read it all in an instant.

"It's a creative visualisation meditation using white light and breathing, for cellular healing imagery that I can integrate into my daily routine."

I felt goose bumps rise on my arms. I sunk back into the overstuffed couch that had been my comfort space since returning from hospital.

Our family's rhodesian ridgeback dog, Max, curled back into his sleeping position, resting against my leg. Max had been so close to me since my mastectomy expedition that I thought our molecules would merge.

Wow this is the missing piece that I have been looking for, I thought excitedly.

'Nine steps' was an amazing book about courage and life saving decisions which dared you to step outside the square. I took the homeopathy medicine and regularly practiced this cellular healing meditation as I imagined that I was watching the white light energy repair my damaged cells. I supplemented my diet with multi vitamins, antioxidants and vitamin C powder. My basic diet consisted mainly of raw vegetables, tuna and fruit to ready my body for healing. I had been advised to avoid micro waved foods, margarine, artificial sweeteners specifically aspartame, sugar and animal fats. The latter two substances were reputed to feed cancer and the former substances were considered to be potentially toxic to the immune

system. The more I meditated the more positive I felt about my future. I felt invigorated, empowered and motivated. I took time out everyday to walk my dogs, enjoy my surroundings and really smell the roses.

I was enjoying my life a day at a time knowing that it wasn't over yet. I still had many hospital visits ahead of me though, where my scar would be checked for healing. There were processes and procedures to follow after a mastectomy and it wasn't long before I was in the hospital clinic's waiting room waiting for my turn for the double appointment with the surgeon followed by an oncology appointment.

I don't know why I have to visit the oncologist, I thought shaking my head in an effort to empty my mind, but the speculative thoughts just kept coming. *Surely the surgeon can tell me what I need to know. That is that they took all the cancer through the mastectomy and that the lymph nodes are clear and that I won't need further intervention or treatment.* I looked around the waiting room where I saw someone, just like me but with her drainage tubes supported in the handmade shoulder bag. She looked pale and frightened. She appeared to be clinging to her friend beside her. I was frightened too but even more frightened by what I just saw.

Well what if the lymph nodes aren't clear then what are you going to do? I know they are because the surgeon told me that the operation was successful. Sighing loudly I chose to change my focus. I imagined that I would visit the coffee shop for a delectable latte. I could smell the coffee bean aroma. I could taste the exquisiteness of the bean and I could feel the warm smooth coffee spill down my throat, warming me from the inside out. I imagined that I could enjoy this latte in between appointments before facing the oncology appointment. Back in the waiting room thoughts bombarded me. I *don't have to worry; the oncology appointment is just a formality. After all most processes have procedures to follow. Yes that is what it is about I assured myself. After all, I remembered at the last clinic appointment, the young intern telling me that it is a normal progression to follow a mastectomy with chemo therapy.*

I rationalised then that I would not fall within the norm, because I knew that they got it all. *There would be nothing left to treat. After all they've taken the whole breast and the operation was successful, my surgeon said so*, I affirmed over and over in my mind.

I continued to sit in the hospital specialist clinic's waiting room for my turn to see my surgeon. I had bought a book to read just in case, I knew that I needed a distraction, but I had forgotten my reading glasses. It was a paper back version of '*The Da Vinci Code*'. If I squinted I could make out the words. Two hours passed when I saw my surgeon walking towards a passageway at the back of the hospital. Maybe it was smoko time. However more time slipped by and he hadn't returned.

He must have had an emergency. I thought, *Well yeh, and saving someone's life was critical and far more important than telling me that I would be fine.* I patiently waited but after more time passed, I couldn't console myself any longer. I felt forgotten and abandoned, especially when I looked around to see that I was the last person in the waiting room and I had the early morning appointment. Once again my stress levels were fuelled with feelings of anxiety, which fired every nerve in my body leading me to feel panic and then anger. Tears were welling in my eyes.

Finally the nurse came to tell me that it was my turn and sure enough a young intern called my name. She was very pleasant and told me that my pathology tests were back.

"I'm ready to hear the results," I said assuring myself that everything would be okay. *Besides I would have been contacted already if anything were truly wrong.*

"Let's look at your surgical site," The young intern said.

"What about my pathology results?" I asked. I wanted confirmation that I was clear of any cancers.

"Okay we will look at those first. The lymph nodes are clear and the tissue around the extracted lump is clear." The young intern said.

I breathed a sigh of relief.

"I won't need chemotherapy then?" I asked confidently.

The young intern said, "Yes you most surely will have to follow with chemo."

I was shocked. I knew instinctively that chemotherapy made no sense. I must have looked ashen because she offered to print a copy of results for me to take home.

"Yes thank you", I said when my mind quickly drifted.

There were always exceptions to the rule, look at the English language it's riddled with exceptions to the rule and I would fall into the exceptions category, I thought.

The specialist nurse made me a cup of tea. "We'll bring your oncology appointment forward so that you can spend some time away from the hospital this afternoon, "she suggested kindly.

"Oh no, but thank you, but oh no my husband Tim won't be here." I blurted. I pulled myself together, telling myself that I'd be fine because I wouldn't need further treatment. What was there to treat? I really wanted Tim to be with me but his work had taken him to the other side of the city, he was too far away. Tim had planned to be there for the late afternoon appointment. I raced outside to turn on my mobile phone to ring him.

"I just need to be positive," I affirmed out loud. "The surgeon probably had an emergency to attend and was possibly saving someone's life." I said into the phone. "I have to go it's my turn to see the Oncologist. The specialist nurse is calling me. Yes, yes, I will be okay Tim, it is just procedure."

The stress of waiting dropped a decibel. I felt a little better. I generated confidence from where I don't know and walked into the consultation room and sat down. The Specialist who would be my Oncologist made a melodramatic entrance, sliding his tall frame into his consultation chair whilst slapping my notes onto his desk top.

"Well where are you going to have your treatment in North Queensland or down here?"

I must have looked confused. The Oncologist continued,

"Well the Pathology results show that you had an invasive aggressive cancer removed. I have decided that you will have an aggressive chemotherapy treatment to ensure it doesn't come back."

I was speechless as I stared at him. The oncologist continued his repertoire,

"A side effect of this chemo treatment is secondary cancer which would present in the bones, brain or the other breast." The rest of his sentence disappeared into the ether as I checked that I was still conscious and not dreaming. My heart was palpitating, sweat was forming all over my body and my head felt like it was full of cotton wool.

Why was I being prescribed a cocktail of aggressive drugs? I thought.

My mind raced back to my post surgical scene in the hospital. I visualised my scene of hope, where I had driven myself to exercise, as soon as possible after my operation to keep the blood flowing and my limbs nimble. I had my own pole, a portable pole fitted to support my lifelines, well my drainage tubes and other stuff that was hanging from me. The pole allowed me mobility to shuffle around the hospital hallways. *I am doing the pole shuffle around the hospital corridors. If I practice I could get better and better every day. I could eventually leave work and make my fortune pole dancing.* I remembered that this thought made me giggle, as I headed back to my ward. I had shuffled down the hallway when I spotted a group of men and women blocking the entrance to my room. I realised that this group was headed by my surgeon. He was much taller than the rest of the group with a shock of black hair back combed which emphasised his larger European forehead and highlighted his serious blue eyes.

"Hello," I said. My Surgeon looked a little bemused.

He doesn't recognise me, I thought.

"You should have taken both," I said as I pulled my T shirt tight across my body. "See now I look lopsided."

My surgeon's jaw dropped, his eyes diverted to my empty bed. He smiled, the muscles around his mouth moved but words were not forthcoming. He extended his arm and ushered me back to my empty bed for examination. When he found his voice he told me that my operation was successful. I interpreted that as the cancer was now behind me. I felt a warm fuzzy feeling sweep over me and through me. Then I pulled my mind back to the present, listening to my Oncologist's speak.

"Statistically you have a 50% chance of survival. Having chemotherapy will increase your survival to 60% if you begin your treatment within six weeks of your mastectomy."

That's 10%, I thought. It was like someone had pressed an on button where I would link 10% with no hope. My mind spun back to a time when I had sat with my baby in my arms opposite an Oncologist in another hospital. I remember how sick my first born son Andrew was through his chemotherapy and radiation treatment. This memory caused my gut to knot, stirring tears to form behind my eyelids pushing hard to spill their way down my cheeks. Guilt consumed me as I remembered Andrew's short life journey. I wished hard to believe that I had tried my best to help Andrew heal. At the time I had felt helpless, especially when Andrew's Oncologist said, "We can cure the cancer that Andrew presents with but we don't know that we can cure Andrew. Honestly, I will give him a 10% chance of survival."

No, its statistics, that's what we were talking about. I can play this game, I thought.

"How long do I have if I do nothing?" I asked quite seriously

"Based on statistics I would say six years," The Oncologist responded. He looked so serious like his eyes were penetrating me from one side of my head through to the other side. I looked away and down at the floor.

Six years, I thought, *I have time to find my own answer. If I choose to have chemo then I won't be able to think straight as I will be too busy looking through a fog into the bottom of a bucket.*

My Oncologist must have read my thoughts as he said, "chemotherapy has come a long way. We also now effectively administer an anti nausea drug with the chemotherapy drugs. In fact I feel heartened when I see my chemotherapy patients bringing sandwiches and drinks to their treatment sessions. I used to watch them come in with just a bucket."

This image scared me. I heard him say bucket and tell me that treatment would take about three months.

My oncologist drew diagrams for me using statistics to illustrate the potential seriousness of this disease that had manifested itself in my body. He told me that based on statistics he knew that the outcome without follow up chemotherapy treatment could potentially prove fatal. My Oncologist seemed to be focusing his attention on me, like he cared for me. He emphasised the *need* for me to act. He was with me, trying to help me battle the big C. I could feel my chest contract, I felt sweat bead around my body, and my mouth was dry, just like the bottom of a very dry gravel pit. Blaming thoughts crept into my mind. I couldn't help thinking that I had unwittingly caused this cancer. My thoughts were morphing into questions. *Why had I taken HRT? Hadn't I heard somewhere that the side effects of taking HRT could be breast cancer? Breast cancer is big and frightening I only had a dehydrated pea sized lump that couldn't possibly cause this much trouble, could it?*

I drifted back to the present again listening to my Oncologist's speak,

"Many more people are now surviving due to follow up chemotherapy treatment. The different variable today is chemotherapy treatment." My Oncologist paused, he focused on me. I felt that he was trying to gauge whether his words had become my knowledge. He took a deep breath and said, "You're a librarian. You can look up the treatment drugs on the internet. I'll write the name of the treatment on a piece of paper for you."

I watched him scribble whilst listening to his continued oration, "I need you to know that historically when tumours were completely removed with a margin of surrounding unaffected tissue it was assumed that the cancer was gone. However research has shown that in circumstances like yours, traces of cancer can be left in the body but often too small to detect. In time this cancer would reappear in a more sophisticated form and kill."

My Oncologist paused waiting for my reaction. Behind my indifferent mask my mind was racing. I felt my head thump and felt my gastric juices rise into my throat. I swallowed and mustered the courage to ask, "You mean that even though there were no identifiable cancer affected cells left in my body there is still a chance, according to research, that there could just be very small stains of cancer cells which would at the moment be so small that they would be unidentifiable using today's technology?" I waited for the Oncologist's response.

He looked at me and nodded, "Yes it could be so small that even the latest scanning technology would not pick it up."

I asked, "Do you think that some cells may have escaped into my bloodstream because of the stirring or the cells during the two biopsies or could the cancer cells have leaked during surgery?"

The Oncologist softened his tone, "Oh no. That would not have happened as a result of surgery."

He took a breath, looked me in the eye and quietly said, "I used to lose sleep when people decided to use only complimentary therapies, but not anymore." I imagined that he held a white flag of surrender.

I needed time to think. In between this noise of my imaginings, questioning thoughts brewed, how could I be smitten with this terrible disease and yet feel better than I had in a long time?

My knowledge was that the surgeon got all the cancer and that the surrounding tissue was clear, as were my harvested lymph nodes. Doubt flooded my mind. *What if a small untraceable infected cell has escaped and is running round my system multiplying quicker than my regular cells?* I thought.

I pondered some more though I'm not sure how logically, What if I do agree to chemotherapy and it doesn't work then I will be faced with years of discomfort. I would rather six years of quality of life where I could function as I do now rather than coping with what I knew of the side effects of chemotherapy.

I finally agreed to think about the Oncologist's advice before committing to a decision. I made an appointment to come back for another consultation with Tim as my support.

There's no way I can do this alone, I thought as I made my way through the hospital corridors to the car park. My thoughts tumbled in my head whilst I tried to make sense of my feelings. These feelings of abandonment and aloneness took me back to when I was seven years old.

When I was seven years old my lifestyle had been stolen from me by a crooked solicitor who I've since referred to as Mr Crook, who through dishonest dealings effectively stole my family's business, my family's home and my life as I knew it. For the latter five years of my seven year life my home was above the café on Main Street below and between the kitchen and the bakery which backed onto the back lane. As long as I could remember this had been my home in this new Australian unfriendly country Victorian town where I lived with my big brothers, big sister and my mum and dad. All of my friends lived off the back lane, above and behind their parents' businesses that serviced their customers and the public on Main Street. My Mum and Dad had built a thriving business that they had planned to sell on the promise of a lengthy lease renewal for the building. I was excited to think that my Mum would have time to spend with me like some of my friends' mums spent with them. I wanted to learn how to cook, and decorate light shades just like my friend next door did with her mum. Selling the business would have meant that my mum would have time to play with me. Mr Crook had verbally promised my Mum and Dad a further seven year lease renewal for their business premises but at the eleventh hour without telling my parents, Mr Crook, signed the lease over to a new shop keeper. I remember that day when my Mum and Dad returned from the Solicitor's meeting. They looked so sad; I thought that they were going to cry. The days following the visit with Mr Crook filled with gloom.

A big fat heavy gloom filled me as my family pulled shop fittings from the walls, discussed how much money they would get if they sold the fridges and other mumblings between the tears. I saw legs stretching and bending as they supported the bodies that were demolishing my world around me. I heard my Dad say, "do something in life to be someone and to have what cannot be taken away from you."

I would no longer be part of the back lane. I somehow understood that Mr Crook had stolen our family business, our family home and my life as I knew it. I felt so helpless, worthless, displaced and disillusioned and I could only watch as the grownups in my world hurt.

My mind jumped to memories of the aftermath of my life's displacement. It seemed that it wasn't enough to lose my home. The following year some higher power beyond my control tried to take my mum too. Early one morning before school my mum had collapsed and was found lying on the floor of the kitchen. I watched the Ambulance Officer wheel my mum into the ambulance to drive her away from me. I remembered the strong sense of having no control of what was happening in my life. I literally watched as feelings of abandonment, inferiority and vulnerability swept through me. I didn't want people to think that I was weak. I didn't like those feelings. I was frightened of feeling just as powerless in the midst of chemotherapy treatment with no hair, skin rashes that itched so much they hurt, uncomfortable infections, mood swings and no energy to walk down the street. In the perception of my world I had seen it all before.

I took a deep breath as I tried to objectively review the situation at hand. I was eating well, much better than I had in years. Excess weight was disappearing and my complexion was radiant, complimenting the copper colour of my short cropped hair. I felt that my sense of inner wellness showed on the outside. I noticed that the people surrounding me in my life were happy to be around me. No one was wearing black or avoiding me because they didn't know what to say. I smiled thinking that all I really needed was a new breast to replace the one taken and I would be complete again.

I found my car in the car park where I had left it only a few hours earlier. The sun was shining and the car's air-conditioning was keeping me cool. I needed time to concentrate and listen to my racing thoughts. *I'm just getting better from the operation and now they want to make me sick again.* Whilst sitting alone in the car I took the opportunity to talk to myself out loud. I said, "I'll go home and think about this quietly. I have to remain positive. I must keep positive. After all that was the one thing that the orthodox and alternative health people with whom I had engaged agreed upon."

I drove into the familiar tree lined driveway. Our dogs Max and Linds were jumping around the car, welcoming me in anticipation of a pat and a bone. I sat on the veranda for a while with the dogs watching as they munched on their bones. It seemed that they were neither contemplating their past nor planning for their future. Max and Linds were free to be totally present with their awareness honed to the demolition of their favourite bone treats. They held them tightly between their front paws whilst they busily salivated and knawed on their big raw bones.

"Enjoy," I said loudly to both dogs. It was time for me to go inside and source some reliable information on FEC chemotherapy treatment.

I followed my Oncologist's suggestion that I check his prescribed chemo brew on the internet. I googled the course of treatment prescribed which led me through authentic medical websites. Amongst the mix I sourced the name of a drug "Adriamycin" a major anticancer drug used frequently in the treatment of many cancers which I remembered was included in my son Andrew's chemotherapy mix. The Adriamycin drug was the one that made Andrew vomit or so I believed. I remembered that Andrew vomited several times a day every day until the chemotherapy treatment stopped. I realised then that I needed to get past this fear of vomiting. No matter how hard I tried to ignore my fear it seemed to grow, causing me to almost feel the vomit creep into my throat burning its way to the outside. My head felt like it was spinning and my limbs seemed to feel like they wanted to collapse. I tried deep breathing like I was taught in my birthing classes. I found that this time I was so busy concentrating on my breathing that my mind emptied, allowing me to be still and relaxed, seducing me into a meditative state.

I relaxed and cleared my mind to just contemplate my future using orthodox chemotherapy medical treatment when a vision just popped onto the movie screen in my mind. I could see a wreath of black tulips on a shiny black coffin decorated with even shinier brass fittings. I was resting peacefully inside, with my arms crossed on my chest, snug within the white satin lining. I could even hear the soft voices that were echoing around my stillness.

"Hey we tried but it didn't work. Anna must be from the minority statistics . . . those who die." I reflexively shifted in my chair when fearful thoughts invaded my meditative stillness, *I don't want to go there yet. I have too much to live for.* I swear that I felt an arm of reassurance embrace me. I was suddenly moved from being in the drama back to watching the drama play out in front of me on my imaginary movie screen. The curtain fell and I sighed with relief. It felt so real when I was lying there listening to the conversation around me, yet somewhat surreal when I watched the scene play out from afar. I felt a wave of calmness envelope me, wash through me and over me.

With eyes wide open I was back in my conscious realm, in my map of my world, perceiving what I believed to be my real world. In my mind I knew that many people were helped by chemotherapy but at this point in time, I decided that I needed to make my own decisions very carefully. Logically I knew that my cancer was sitting in the kidney dish somewhere, gone from my body. My mini me was reminding me that I didn't want the big C to return.

Intuitively I believed that I knew I could take control of my cancer journey, I just needed to find the how.

Okay, I thought, *I will just put it out there. I will be open minded and be present to whatever opportunity comes my way.*

Attending the upcoming local cancer support group seemed to be a logical and resourceful step forward. The support group had already helped me with providing someone to talk with me about my cancer experience. They had provided me with written information about breast cancer and given me a handmade shoulder bag to hold my post operative attached drainage bottles. There was also a protective thin pillow in my pack for me to use on my car trip home. The pillow would sit under the seatbelt and across my chest to protect the surgical area.

CHAPTER FIVE

"I was advised that I have to have protected sex for six days after chemotherapy treatment," Linda said. Linda was the youngest attendee at the breast cancer support group and seemed to be the only one who was part way through her treatment. Everyone else had hair on their heads and differing shades of colour in their faces. Linda continued, "I thought that there would be others here who would have lost their hair."

I joined the conversation.

"What treatment are you having?" I asked.

"It's an aggressive one that they call FEC", she responded. "I knew that I would lose my hair and I'm supposed to feel sick but fortunately that isn't the case. I'm doing well but my veins aren't doing so well. They couldn't administer the chemotherapy intravenously last time," Linda said.

Just like with Andrew when his chemo was administered in the vein bulging in his head because he was crying so hard. A thought that left me feeling distressed.

"I've got to go. See you next time," I said politely and left.

I left the breast cancer support group session with a directory and guide to breast prostheses and bra fittings after breast surgery.

"That part was good. I won't have to hide my chest by crossing my arm over my chest to hide my body's imbalance. I won't have to feel self conscious any more." I said to the car park empty of people, "I'm not sure about chemotherapy treatment though. Linda is very brave. I don't think that I am brave enough to take that road."

I remembered how very sick Andrew was when he was undergoing chemotherapy. He threw up several times each day. I could relate. I remember my first return trip to the outer Great Barrier Reef where for two hours I clung so hard to the nearest pole on the boat that my molecules almost merged with the boat's timber. I threw up uncontrollably. I remembered that someone had asked me if I was okay.

"Yes," I whined, "Just leave me alone."

It seemed like each word uttered brought my insides to meet the outside world. I had felt all alone in this world, just me, my nausea and the boat's pole that I clutched. It was like the rest of the world existed only in my imagination. I wasn't going to choose to feel like that again because of medical intervention that I believed I could possibly avoid. No matter how hard I tried I couldn't shake the memory of the wretchedness of that nausea feeling. I had felt helpless and out of control. I didn't like feeling out of control. I felt a strong need to take control, to believe and have faith that I could make an alternative decision for my future survival. Nevertheless, I felt compelled to attend a return visit to the Oncologist with Tim the following week, because I said I would. Time was racing by and I needed clarity and certainty that I would make the right decision for me.

I was focusing on finding a way towards an outcome of survival without chemotherapy treatment. Synchronicity was unleashed. It was serendipitous that a friend from the past returned a call in answer to my query regarding a safety incident that involved my children at the local swimming pool. He recommended that I read *The Power of Now,* by Eckart Tolle.

"Our local library has a copy. Go borrow it from them." He advised.

I learned from the library staff that before *The Power of Now* he was recommending that people read *The Journey,* by Brandon Bays. I left the local library with a copy of The *Power of Now* tucked under my arm and a request placed for Brandon Bay's *The Journey.* I realised then that if you ask then there is help out there from the least expected places.

My second appointment with the Oncologist rolled around very quickly. This time I was prepared for a long wait. I had remembered to take my glasses but this time I didn't have to wait too long. The Oncologist welcomed us into his room and then fell into his chair banging the closed file on his desk.

"Well." he said watching me intensely, "What have you decided?"

I felt vulnerable. I felt like I was letting him down. I really liked him. I felt nervous about telling him that I was not going to comply with the orthodox chemotherapy treatment. I could feel my heart race and my breathing was rapid. I didn't know whether I would be able to stick by my decision to tell him that I wasn't going down the chemotherapy path. My fearful emotions were all encompassing when I thought about chemotherapy. I interrupted my emotions when I perceived how incongruous it was to me that my Oncologist was of Chinese origin with a Russian name. I was tempted to laugh at my crazy notion that he was different to my stereotyping of people's names. I noticed that my heart rate and my breathing had slowed. I actually felt a calm feeling arise within me. I sat up straight in my chair feeling confident that I could choose what I believed to be best for me over what would please others. I reminded myself that I needed to take control of my life and my decisions. I didn't have to base my decision on pleasing the Oncologist. After all it wasn't like I was back at school, obliged to sit before the headmistress whilst being reprimanded for something that I did or didn't do. I was conditioned and had learned well to be subservient. I was about to break that pattern and make one of the hardest decisions in my life, to tell an authorative figure that I wasn't going to do abide by his decision for me.

I looked the Oncologist in the eye and quietly almost sheepishly said,

"Well I think that I will go alternative."

I could do with some assertiveness training here, I chided myself.

Thank God for my husband Tim as he quickly took up the challenge to support me. The Oncologist responded very well to Tim, answering the many questions that were thrown his way. I managed to break into the conversation at times with questions of my own. At one point I even tried to bargain with the Oncologist telling him that I would prefer not to use chemo this time, but if there were to be a next time then I would go with chemotherapy treatment.

"If it comes back then it will probably hit the receptors and be chemo resistant so there would be nothing that we could do," The Oncologist said. Now I understood his angst. The Oncologist turned to Tim and said,

"Medicine has come a long way. For example your son Andrew's undifferentiated sarcoma proved to be chemo resistant. In today's medicine Andrew would be given stem cell treatment, well that is of course if they could find a compatible cord. Stem cell treatment just wasn't available twenty years ago."

My mind went into overdrive. I had followed Doctor's orders then and let Andrew be administered with chemotherapy. My thoughts raced back in time. Chemotherapy made Andrew so sick that his faeces literally burnt him when he evacuated. He suffered all of this even though his illness was chemo resistant. Andrew's Oncology team were planning to keep Andrew on chemotherapy for two years, had he survived. I nearly cried thinking that I had allowed Andrew's ineffective treatment that caused him so much pain. My stomach churned, my head felt like it was stuffed with cottonwool and my chest filled with air. I exhaled with a sigh. *How could they have given my little boy chemotherapy for chemo resistant cancer?* I thought angrily, *and now they want me to undergo chemotherapy treatment just in case there is a tiny spec of cancer waiting to implode within me.* In my opinion I made it mean that it made no sense. I took a deep breath and directed my attention back into the room.

I just have to sit here a little longer, I thought to myself.

Not giving up the Oncologist looked me in the eye, sat back in his chair and drew breath.

"Now I have told you what we can offer you. Tell me what you plan as an alternative."

I felt like I was competing to win just like I had at school when I competed in athletics or netball and I was not going to let him beat me. I haemorrhaged information about positive thinking, meditation, eating well, supplementing with vitamins and minerals. I had some knowledge that I was able to embellish.

"Well I'm going to eat appropriately, use meditation and creative visualisation and um take supplements including vitamin C, selenium and anti-oxidants. When our son was sick we had pathology tests that showed a lack of selenium and vitamin C"

I didn't let on that I had lots of ideas but just a sniff of a road to follow. Just like the example in the secret where the car shines its lights at night to illuminate the path ahead and that is as far as we can see. We travel beyond the lights because we have faith that we will get to our destination. My faith was wavering. I certainly didn't tell my Oncologist how scared I felt. There was a pregnant pause, followed by a carefully enunciated sentence,

"Well alternative medicine didn't save your son." The Oncologist said earnestly.

I reacted uncontrollably, "Well neither did chemotherapy."

I could feel blood rush through my body making every nerve in my body prickle. I was angry that Andrew hadn't been saved. I needed to calm down and respond to this man sitting in front of me who was sharing his expertise to give me the best chance that he knew how to give for me to have longevity. We sat in silence for a while and then I said that I would give some thought to using chemotherapy and complementary medicine together. Tim and I left the hospital quietly we didn't speak until we got into the car.

Driving away from the hospital Tim and I agreed to grab a cup of coffee from our favourite coffee shop in the mall. The car was on automatic pilot heading in the direction towards the coffee shop anyway.

We burrowed into a quiet cosy corner of an almost empty coffee shop. The coffee was soothing and the delicious chocolate covered cake melted in our mouths. We had our fill of delectable delicacies and we were cocooned in our own safe part of the world where we watched the few people left in the shopping centre go about their business. Life around us continued. People around us were seemingly totally oblivious to us and what was happening to us. Our environment's energy was indifferent clearing the way for me to think.

"You know Tim, for the first time in my life I know that I am making the right decision. I am not going down the chemotherapy path. Usually my mind plagues me with doubts when I make decisions. This is the first time I can remember that I have made a definite decision without a doubt.

This is what it must feel like to be in control of your life." I stopped for breath, bathing in my feelings of empowerment and contentment. This must be the feeling that people have who believe that they can do anything. In my excitement words spilled from my mouth,

"I believe that I can do this alternative healing on my own but it would be good to be part of a support group of the same ilk. You know my friend Chris who I used to work with at my previous job has the right connections to new age practice. I know she has the knowledge. I got a Xmas card from Chris with her new phone number on it. I'll call her when I get home. I can do this I know I can." We both smiled.

Tim and I sat a little longer draining our coffee cups whilst chatting about our boys and whiling away the time watching the world go by. Finally our cups were emptied. The white porcelain lining on the inside of my empty cup shined. There was no coffee left to drink. It was time for us to walk out of the coffee shop and into the immense space of the almost empty shopping mall.

"Hey there's Chris," Tim said.

"Yeh right," I mumbled.

I looked to where Tim was pointing and there she was, her long blonde hair neatly brushed, contrasting with her navy business jacket. Chris was waiting to meet with someone, her teenage son I think.

"I've been trying to find you" Chris said excitedly," There's a *Journey* seminar tomorrow and Sunday. I heard that you were in town and I'd like you to come."

I was blown away so to speak that she had thought of me and was inviting me to join her. Chris drew breath and continued," It's about peeling back the layers of emotions to clear and change cellular memories using the guided journey processes to heal."

Chris's description of '*The Journey*' sounded familiar, it sounded like the processes that I had read from, *'Nine steps to reversing or preventing cancer and other diseases/learn to heal from within'*, by Shivani Goodman. *Wow it was like someone up there likes me because now I have the opportunity to learn 'the how 'in the way that I learn best through participation and learning the steps.*

"Yes I'd love to join you," I said.

Saying yes to Chris felt good like it was the next small step that I needed to take towards feeling that I was resourcefully taking control of my life and my life's ultimate outcome. I felt a deep gratitude for a wonderful gift of being valued and gift of hope.

"You know Chris. This is a God thing meeting like this." We smiled knowingly then we hugged, and said our goodbyes.

CHAPTER SIX

A split second decision to embrace an opportunity to attend a weekend workshop empowered me to choose to believe that I would contribute to changing my cellular memories, to heal, through experiencing Brandon Bay's *Journey* work.

There must be at least three hundred people here, I thought. I was surrounded by people, mainly women. I could see the odd male dotted here and there in the audience.

In my perception of my map of my world or in my opinion this *Journey Intensive* seminar was not only filling the gaps of the how for my personal healing journey, it was also helping me to uncover cellular memories and find the origins of my limiting beliefs that were influencing my life today. I learned that our cells are continuously regenerating themselves, with old cells being replaced by new cells. For some reason the new cells carried across the memories in the old cells. I learnt to be a time traveller going back in time to discover a different reality around what I had perceived as the reality in my memories. I discovered that Andrew's Oncologist was doing the best he could to heal Andrew with the resources that he had. I had forgotten that I trusted that he was doing his best to help Andrew.

Journey work reminded me of a large part of the Silva method that I thought that I had forgotten. I had participated in the Silva mind control method training out of curiosity. I had taken from it what was relevant to my life at the time. The Silva relaxation techniques allowed me to break the rhythm of stress that happened through living my life by reacting to life instead of responding to it. It seemed to me that immersing myself in journey work would empower me and give me the courage to know that I could discover, change and heal my cellular memories to change my beliefs and attitudes to serve me better. Brandon Bays writes about her experience of self healing from cancer without medical intervention. José Silva, the self-taught psychologist and founder of the world-renowned Silva Method promoted Mind Body Healing, where he investigated the mind's extraordinary control over your physical body. I thought about one of Andrew's Doctors who told me so long ago that he had seen cancers reduce in his patients when people prayed for them and then when the praying stopped the cancer would regrow. Just thinking about that gave me hope, excitement even. In my younger years I had felt helpless and believed that life just happened to you. I guess I had been given some control knowing that if you were good then you would go to heaven and if you were bad you would go to hell. I just never knew what good and bad meant or how I was supposed to be good.

My fear of what could be if I didn't have chemotherapy treatment as prescribed encouraged me to find change. I remembered my Oncologist telling me that if I continued to do what I do then based on statistics cancer would return even more destructively. I was afraid of dying but more so afraid of spending eternity unpleasantly because I carried an embedded belief that I wasn't good enough for the gold lined streets of heaven. Whilst I was breathing I didn't have to think about it so I needed to continue to breath. I would need to consciously take responsibility for my own life because honestly chemotherapy for me was just as scary as dying because I understood that it didn't come with a guarantee of living a long life where I could continue ignoring my greatest fear through that belief that I wasn't good enough.

Through Journey work I would shake that belief that I was destined to unpleasant places in eternity because I wasn't meeting the measures which I didn't understand anyway. I would change my beliefs through self discovery and self awareness where I would learn about me and my experiences that had formed those beliefs that had moulded me into the person that I had become. Through Journey work processes I realised that

I could set goals through inspiration rather than through desperation, I could take control of my life. I felt like I had found the pot of gold at the end of the rainbow. I was beginning to really understand and believe that I have the resources within me to change my life. I had learned that through the Silva mind method too, though at the time I had not taken that extra step to make my learnings my knowledge. There was so much to learn and I was discovering that this rabbit hole of learning and growing self awareness was deep and I felt like I was only brushing the surface.

Through the Journey processes I had learned to uncover my defining moments that had become my cellular memories which were deeply entrenched. A major defining moment in my life was when I imagined that I travelled back in time where my life as I knew it at seven years of age had been taken by Mr Crook. This memory had embedded itself in my cells where I would play the pattern of fearing that I was not good enough, that I didn't belong, that I was abandoned and that I was unloved. Going back in time I discovered that I reacted with feelings of helplessness, bewilderment and the fear of abandonment. This was a pattern that I would play out in other experiences in my life. When I was ten years old my life of freedom as I had known it in country Victoria had been taken away from me when we moved to the restrictive rules of city living where I just didn't fit in. I was widowed at twenty two years of age leaving me to feel guilty and abandoned. At thirty years of age my first born son was taken from me just before his first birthday leaving me with a feeling of helplessness and sadness because I couldn't help him get better. Through Journey work I felt that I had finally grasped the how of transforming my negative emotions and fears around my life that impacted on my health to take responsibility for my decisions and ultimately take control of my health. I learnt this by imagining that I was moving through layers of the build up of emotions, to the void and then through the void to those pleasant emotions where I became aware of a me that was buried way below the layers of limiting beliefs and helpless attitudes that were bearing down on me and suffocating who I am.

It was an amazing experience to discover where my embedded beliefs had come from. I found that my memories were distorted and that I had deleted the good things around those bad memories. Just like I had focused on the trauma of my son Andrew's life instead of focusing on the gift of love from having a special child in my life, having said that I do believe that all children are special in their own unique ways. I loved how we learned that we can go back in time and change our beliefs to change how we feel and change our attitudes around who we are being.

Let me tell you about this one guy in my life. When I met him and for a couple of years later he was my friend until he changed and then every time I saw him after that he would make my skin crawl. In my map of my world I saw that he was as slippery as a snake sliding through olive oil. I learned that it was my resentment towards him that caused me to visualise him that way. I went through the journey process of revisiting our friendship. I believed he was my friend and then one day he tricked me into trusting him as a friend. I had confided in him that I thought his stress could have been triggered by a bully whom we both knew. He told the bully, became friends with the bully and I was moved on. I made a belief around that he feigned friendship with me to use my information to align with the bully for his benefit so that I would be moved on and not him. Going back in time, I realised then that he was petrified of change. Through his underhandedness I had missed out and was moved on. When I revisited the experience I realised that I had in fact moved away from the bullying environment and then I moved toward something much better. In my mind he had inadvertently done me a huge favour. He was stuck in a bullying environment and I was free or at least that is how I felt. I went through a process in my mind of forgiving him. When I saw him again I felt an indifference towards him. He didn't make my skin crawl anymore he was just another person on the face of the earth. When it suited me I would choose to respond to him with a hello when I saw him. I changed my belief around him. I was almost grateful that he had chosen to stay in the bullying environment instead of me. He had saved me and let me free. The thought warmed me from the inside. Of course I was grateful I had that warm fuzzy feeling of freedom. If I could choose to change my feelings and my attitude towards people around me, I could change how I lived my life. *Yes I could use my inner resources to choose to live large, choose courageously and choose to live without limits. I could possibly choose to change my mind and change my body, to feel better and be better and better. I somehow felt lighter and the world outside was brighter. I could do this, I could take control, I could change my beliefs and attitudes to change my life and change my health.*

Through previous counselling I had uncovered that in the past I didn't even give myself permission to deal with big stuff that happened in my life.

"It sounds like you haven't dealt with your son's passing," said a counsellor to me during a work related team building workshop some years earlier. This middle aged appropriately qualified psychologist stirred questions within me. I asked, "Okay, but how do I deal with it or know that I have dealt with it?"

At that time Andrew's memory constantly brought tears to my eyes. She had observed my reactions.

"Make an appointment and we will work through it," The psychologist suggested kindly.

I knew I needed help when Andrew died but I didn't know how to ask for it or where to get it from. Andrew's Oncologist Doctor wasn't even at the hospital when he died. I decided at that time to believe that Andrew's Oncologist only came to see me because he needed to negotiate approval from Tim and me to perform a post mortem on Andrew's body not to support us through this last bit of our experience. I didn't consider every other family in the hospital that he looked after I was just thinking of us.

Andrew's Oncologist said, "Like Andrew, a three year old boy has presented with the same rare tumour. If we do a post mortem on Andrew's body we may find something to help this boy, though we may find nothing."

Tim and I agreed to allow a post-mortem. Then I remember feeling alone even though I was supported and surrounded by family and friends. I felt like I was being pushed to get over Andrew's death and get on with my life.

Through the first emotional journey process I learned that I hadn't realised that I was in fact the one pushing. I was not allowing me time for the grievance processes, nor had I given myself permission to ask for help. I believed that I would prove to the world that I could rely on me to be strong. I discovered sadness within me a sadness that had lingered for 21 years.

My very first Journey emotional process demonstrated to me that I had indeed not dealt with or had closure of my son Andrew's death from cancer. I learned through the *journey* process to welcome my pain, where I cried heaps and released that pain through forgiveness. I was filled with gratitude to have the opportunity to finally realise that I had worked towards closure.

Closure for me meant that I could appreciate and value the time that I had with Andrew. My tears changed from tears of sadness for Andrew's pain and my loss of a son, to tears of joy remembering the love we shared and tears of gratitude to have been his mother albeit for less than one year. I had discovered an awareness of life's special gift to me. My little man would live with me forever reminding me of his gift to me of love and trust. Andrew's passing had transformed from the tragedy of death and loss to the celebration of my brave little man's life.

Brandon Bay's teachings gave me the how for forgiveness, gratitude and appreciation. I had discovered a process that I could use to identify my defining moments that created my embedded beliefs that influenced my behaviour. Using my imagination I would travel back through time to see what really happened around my defining moments. Expanding my awareness of the moment changed my attitude towards uncovered issues. Through the journey processes I allowed myself time to reflect and see what really happened. I would forgive where I needed to forgive and appreciate with gratitude for what I had gained. I found that after the processes I could feel my emotions shift turning those toxic stressful feelings that weighed me down to a much lighter happier feeling. I have learned that stress typically describes a negative concept that can have an impact on one's mental and physical well-being. The beyond blue website says that stress makes your body produce chemicals that raise your heart rate and blood pressure and increase mental focus. This helps you to perform well in a challenging situation over a short period of time. The problems from stress happen when stress is regular and doesn't let up. The chemicals the body releases can build up and cause changes that damage your physical and mental health. On the second day of the Journey intensive seminar I experienced my very first Journey physical healing process. I visualised a pulsating red circle surrounded by a darker red ring. It was near my heart, close to the area where that ductal carcinoma lump had appeared. I could feel my heart race. I panicked thinking that this was the cancer regrowing like my Oncologist talked about. I pushed this thought from my awareness and continued to trust the process. Once again Andrew's illness featured in my visualisations.

Through the physical journey process I created a safe and protected space in my imagination where I was able to seek closure. I had an awareness that children are only ever on loan to their parents and the time with them is to be cherished. I needed closure of the red hole that was so close to my heart. It was like I needed to mend the hole that Andrew's passing had left in my heart. Towards the end of the process, in my visualisation I realised that the hole was from the recently removed drainage tube that still needed to heal. That hole had served its purpose for me and would heal. It was not a cancerous growth that I was dealing with at all. I felt awareness, even a certainty around my life that I really would be getting better and better every day in every way. Immediately after the physical process work I could actually feel the pain in my side lessen. I sat quietly in the deep plush conference room chairs when an older lady with short grey hair approached me. "Are you okay?" she asked.

"Yes I'm just sitting, contemplating for a moment," I responded.

The older lady burst into a huge smile. She was so excited to tell me,

"I have just qualified as a *Journey* Practitioner. I've been accepted for placement in Africa to be part of the *Journey* team where I will be helping kids and others." She stopped for breath and then asked, "Can I get you a cup of tea?"

"Thank you for your offer but I have a glass of water," I replied.

Wow, I thought, *her excitement is infectious. How exciting would it be to get to that point in your life where you have grown so much that you can lovingly contribute to those in need in such a big way.*

I left '*the Journey*' intensive workshop with recorded CD's of the emotional and physical process work which included the healing sands meditation for me to use at home. Every night I listened to my healing sands meditation C.D. inducing me to sleep peacefully. I continued to work through the processes to grow my self awareness around who I really am and understand why this cancer and other life experiences happened to me. I was beginning to see my breast cancer experience as a gift which would potentially transform into the best personal growth journey of my life.

I had so far discovered that I had carried an attitude of accepting the blame for others feelings and totally ignoring my own. When I was four years old I was chased and beaten by a neighbour's mother because in her mind I had upset her son. I had reacted to his taunts, we had a fight and he lost. I didn't do it again for fear of being beaten by his mother. I made this mean that he was more important than me.I had accepted her judgement of him being more important than me. I took this young child's taunts, sacrificing my feelings to ensure that his were intact. I discovered that I innately felt undeserving of being loved and that the perception of my destiny was to be a cog in a wheel rather than an individual person.

Through religious speak I was told that I was born a sinner and would be punished. It was only the chosen righteous few who would escape this punishment. Nobody told me how to be righteous in a way that I understood. Consequently I lived in fear of the punishment. When I was ten years of age I was still having nightmares about that scary place called hell, where I believed I was doomed to spend eternity. If I tried to please everyone else and let everyone else make my decisions for me then surely I would stand a bit of a chance of going to that other place much higher up.

Through self talk I had convinced myself that I was a follower and not a leader. I began to believe that people had a right to control me and it was my duty to please them. As a teenager I continued to go to church with my parents because that was the right thing to do and that would make them happy.

From a teenage peer group perspective I forced myself to learn to smoke cigarettes because it was cool amongst the in crowd. I let others decide how I would be entertained. When asked the question, "What would you like to do?" I had no clue because I let my friends and peer group make those decisions for me. I wanted them to like me and value me. It didn't occur to me that I needed to like me and value me first.

Through the Journey processes I learned about the importance for me of forgiveness. Forgiving me and forgiving others changed my feelings. I would notice releases of energy, often replaced with a peaceful feeling or joyful feelings after each process. To get there I had worked through emotional experiences where I cried, where my heart raced, and where I felt like I was living in a black hole with a heavy feeling which would weigh heavily on my shoulders, back and neck. Sometimes my head ached and I had low energy, until I flipped these feelings within me to a lighter energy, through the Journey processes.

Through the journey processes I discovered beliefs about me like, who was I to think that I could heal myself? I had been inadvertently conditioned, I believed, by my parent's religious belief to think less of myself. Mum had insisted that her religious laws guided her to tell me as her forefathers were guided to tell her that we were all born sinners. I interpreted sinner to mean that I was born into badness, and that I was a bad person. My understanding was that I couldn't escape the badness. I would have to be saved. I didn't really understand what bad and badness was only that is was the opposite of good. The opposite to being saved to live eternity in a wonderful place called Heaven. I remember something about pearly gates and the gold lined streets being the reward for living in heaven. I just wanted to feel good, have self worth, and the confidence to know that I was just as good as the next person.

My perception of my mum's belief was that you were simply chosen to go to heaven. I remember my mum telling me that you had to be good enough to be chosen and while you were waiting to be good enough you could strengthen your chances of going to heaven if you abided by the rules she had learnt from her religion. That was my chunk of understanding of my mum's beliefs. I discovered that I made that chunk of belief mean that I was not good enough. The idea of frying in hell with some evil overseer making my afterlife unbearable scared me too. I wanted to escape that image of burning in hell. When travelling back along my timeline to view my earliest memory of my mum's teachings I realised that my mum was trying to protect me from an eternity of hellfire and damnation. Her intentions were well meaning and good. In fact I learned that my parents were doing the best they could with the resources that they had within them. I discovered that my mum and dad were doing their best to guide me away from the sinners' pain towards freedom and happiness as they knew it to be. I discovered those beliefs that were built on my perception of my parents' teachings. So deeply entrenched were those beliefs that I was too frightened to even question them.

When I was six years old I used to watch my peers breaking these religious laws. Before Church on a Sunday they would cross the road from the Church to spend their collection money on lollies from the local milk bar. I was in awe of this practice. In my mind they dared to tempt the wrath of God by causing others to work on the Sabbath. I did think it strange that they didn't burst into flames in fact nothing happened to them. I would watch them Sunday after Sunday doing the same thing but I never found the courage to do the same. I knew that Sunday was the Sabbath and you were not allowed to work or cause others to work. Buying lollies from the milk bar caused the milk bar owner to work by serving the kids taking their church money in exchange for lollies. Other kids could get away with it but I would burn, I just knew it. These embedded beliefs haunted me and continued to directly affect my life choices. I drew back from my first job opportunity when leaving school because I would have been rostered to work on a Sunday. It was my first job interview that began well and finished badly, when I realised Sunday work was involved it was like my energy was drained from me. I was so afraid of judgement and the punishment of not being good enough besides I lived at home with my Mum and Dad. They would find out and I couldn't see them letting me take a job where I had to work on a Sunday.

Journey work bought to life for me the resources that I already had within me to choose to make changes in my life and my Oncologist had prescribed change for my health success. In my mind's eye it was a win win situation. Through journeywork I was motivated to develop and use my internal resources to take action. Adding journey work to the Silva mind method skills that I had already learned resonated strongly with my needs to take the steps that I needed to take towards my ultimate outcome of taking control of my life. Through my journey I would discover so much about my life, the people in my life those who impact my life and me. I discovered that the more beliefs I changed and emotions I flipped the more there was to change and shift.

CHAPTER SEVEN

"You can go home and put it all behind you and get on with the rest of your life," my G.P. said. He showed me the letter that he had received from the hospital telling him that all went well with my mastectomy.

I stared at him, took a deep breath and told him that I had decided not to take chemotherapy treatment. I closed my eyes expecting the world to fall in around me. I had got into so much trouble from another GP before when choosing to cease Andrew's chemotherapy treatment. I was listening and to my amazement this is what I heard.

"Your prognosis is founded on probability based on statistics," he said with his head buried in his notes about me whilst he annotated. I felt relieved but at the same time the thoughts inside my head raced. I expected to be in trouble for not agreeing to pursue traditional treatments. There was a moment's silence. My G.P. proceeded to tell me that a female friend of his had survived bowel cancer and enjoyed good health in the Coastal Hinterland. He told me how she grew her own vegetables making certain that she ate well to maintain her good health.

"Like her you could go home and grow tomatoes," He continued to say," At least that way you will know that the tomatoes will truly be good for you and they would really be filled with vitamin C and they will taste good too."

I smiled. I felt grateful to be encouraged and not judged. I was six weeks into my recovery phase, past the point of effective chemotherapy treatment anyway. I was feeling better with each passing day. Thoughts were racing around my mind. I stopped one thought and focussed on it.

Why does it worry me what my GP thinks or that he judges me? Afterall I know that some people had called me brave and some people thought that I was foolish but deep in my heart I knew without a doubt that I had made the right decision for me. My GP, he didn't judge me. I could feel a smile creep into my being. I began to think that maybe I had imagined that people were always judging me. The pain of judgement was real and I did try to please everyone at my expense at times but this time I had stood up for myself, stood up for what I believed to be my truth.

Through the journey processes I would discover how powerful it is to open into even my deepest pain, to then find the peace that lies beyond that pain in the very core of my being. I found already that when I processed I felt like I was emptying a bucket full of my past painful experiences, whilst uncovering cellular memories that would be healed and changed through forgiveness and gratitude. I had already experienced the wonder, the magic of the healing power of forgiveness which would be my journey towards healing my mind and my body. I had bucket loads of experience and conditioning to deal with beginning from my very beginning. A beginning that was moulded with generational conditioning and experiences effecting the person that I was conditioned to believe that I was growing into.

I perceived that I was born into a deeply Protestant fundamentalist religious world where generations of people were conditioned to believe that they were born sinners. It never entered my mind to refuse to go to church, even though I so envied my peers who weren't forced to go to church.

I was the newest in my family line to be conditioned to believe that righteous living mixed with belief, repentance and attaining forgiveness for one's life sins would lead me to eternal life in the gold lined walls of heaven. I was scared of my eternal punishment if I failed to become one of the chosen few. Hellfire and damnation were just words but they instilled the greatest fear within me.

From my earliest memories my life was veiled with seriousness. In the strictness of the religious construct there would be no sinful fun activities for me like dancing, partying or watching movies. As a little girl I so wanted to learn to tap dance but I wasn't allowed. This was somehow sinful how I never really understood. I would sneak into dancing sessions with friends who participated and just sit with their mothers and watch. My mum thought that I was playing in my friends' houses. My family's religious history was passed onto me. It was my understanding that some of the strictest members of my extended family professed the belief and conditioned religious followers to believe that make up, short hair and certain clothes were for those bad ladies of the night. It was constantly reinforced that if you dressed like a lady of the night and your language was interpreted as blasphemous your chances of eternal life in heaven were spaced even further away. It was like an epiphany for me to discover that my ancestors' lives were moulded by tradition, guided by strict moral and religious laws which they didn't appear to question. In my mind I questioned and felt that this fundamentalist religion held a destructive judgemental power base of fear for me.

It seemed to me that radical change appeared to challenge my ancestor's religious beliefs, for example, when my grandfather was holding my sister's hand whilst looking skywards watching one of the first planes fly by, he said to Sjanie, "You know it is a sin to fly. If humans were meant to fly then God would have given us wings."

My own life was founded on generation upon generation of social constructs framed by religious beliefs, and moral conditioning. It was like this foundation was attracting more of the same for me. My parents were really strict, enforcing their strange ways on my life. None of my friends had to obey the laws of the Sabbath where I was not allowed to work or cause others to work. I was forced to go to church twice on a Sunday. I was not allowed to study or play sport on a Sunday. My Dutch relations who lived in Holland even frowned upon my friendships with Catholic people, who it seemed, were the opposition. When I was in fourth grade I remember that my mum almost hyperventilated when I told her that I liked the three dimensional coloured illustrations in my friends catholic bible more than the one dimensional black and white etchings in our

Protestant family bible. I told her that I thought it cool that Jesus' blue eyes followed me around the room.

I was so entrenched in my family's strict religious ways that I swear I attracted more of it. How unlucky could I be to be zoned for one of the strictest girls' secondary schools in the universe, governed by the scary headmistress that we called Black Mac? Then on top of that, in my first year of high school my parents found what they believed was a more suitable church for the family to attend. An Irish reformed Presbyterian church with its fundamentalism sitting closely with the fundamental teachings and doctrines as I understood them of the old country's Dutch reformed Presbyterian Church. I so longed to flee this life and flee this life I did building on my experiences at a frenetic pace. Like cancer my bucket loads of experience multiplied faster and faster than my life progressed, giving me so much to process for my mind, body emotional and health journey.

I have learned through my neuro linguistic programming training with Robb Whitewood that our journey in life is about travelling from the present to the future passing goal posts on the way. The vehicle we use to get there is the methodology of travel for our journey. "The vehicle is frequently inherited from family, friends, cultures, socio-economics or religion. Some people choose to walk, others run, and others just drive. It can be of course be traded in at any time you choose." I discovered through my Journey processes that I can go back in time along my timeline to uncover my vehicle's defining moments and embedded beliefs to understand what really happened and then change how I reacted to those moments to change my beliefs through changing the energy that governs my molecules that make my cells which combine to make my organs that make my body work. Just like practicing meditation has been effectively used to reduce the nausea feeling from chemotherapy treatments, breathing techniques are taught for the birthing process to change energy to calming energy. I have gone back in time to discover my defining moments that I have inherited and experienced in my vehicle of life so that I can change the energy to change those cellular memories that don't serve me and choose new beliefs and keep those that serve me.

CHAPTER EIGHT

Kees and Sitje, my Dad and my Mum were married in the late 1930's. Kees was a tall dark and handsome young man. Although he took his responsibilities seriously, he loved to have fun. In some ways he was always a boy at heart. At his funeral he was described as a man with a larrikin streak. My mum was an attractive young lady with a slight build, blue eyes and a rounded face. Sitje was shorter than Kees, though she stood tall when her loyalty and sense of being right was called upon. Kees and Sitje lived in a small country town called Hansweert in the province of Zeeland in the south of the Netherlands. They lived in the family home where Kees was born in 1907. Across the road from Kees and Sitje's home was a dyke wall protecting the land from the sea. The sea level behind the dyke walls was higher than the land below where Kees and Sitje's home and business lay. This particular dyke wall was one of two which lined the waterway with its sluices to control the water levels for incoming boats, essentially providing the boats with safe entrance into other major water ways of Europe. Water seemed to be a commonality between my mum and dad. Sitje's family were connected to the water through their family business. My mum often told me stories of her life living on a barge which travelled the waterways of Holland and Germany. I too loved the water. I loved to swim and scuba dive, for that I am grateful.

Kees developed a fear of water in his first decade of life when he became trapped in water well under the family home, where he nearly drowned. He feared it so much that he couldn't watch me swim. That one time when he did watch me swim he freaked out when I duck dived into the water he frantically asked mum where I was. I was his baby and his youngest child.

Sitje had retained her love of water even though she was forced from it at the tender age of eight because her religious etiquette said that she was getting to old to show her body in a swim suit. It was as though my mum had passed on this love of water to me. In my younger days I would swim in swimming pools, in dams, creeks and the sea regardless of the weather. I later learned to scuba dive where I had a taste of an awesome world in my own magical space. To get there I had pushed through the barriers of my comfort zone to don the scuba diving gear that allowed me to breath underwater where this magic happened. The scuba gear contained me in my own small space within the expansiveness of the ocean from where I could detach and observe the world around me. It seemed that under the water I was free to be me in the safety of the sea. The sea seemed to envelope me, flow through me and infinitely extend me in its expansiveness. I felt protected and confident with my learned knowledge of survival techniques where I could breathe underwater through my regulator and scuba tank, where I could keep myself warm in my wetsuit and keep safe with my scuba instruments. Under the water I was free to observe and watch fish and other scuba divers who were encased in their own bit of space. We were only connected by the surrounding mass of water stretching all around as far as I could see. Being under the water was an escape from judgement and my perception of the social imposed boundaries on land, where values like the 'have's' and 'have not' affected who I was, where I lived and where I fitted in the fabric of life. On land there were often times where I felt that I didn't fit in. Maybe I was meant to be a dolphin, life seemed simpler under water, or maybe I needed to get over myself and somehow capture this same feeling of freedom on land. Through my map of the world I perceived that it was different for my Mum and Dad.

Both my parents' families were financially comfortable to the point that neither my Mum nor Dad were even aware of the lifestyle change and financial hardships that people faced during the depression in the 1930's.

Kees and Sitje's families were able to continue to tithe their earnings to the church. They even had enough money to continue paying for their expensive church seats. Apparently in those days where you sat in church reflected where you stood in society.

Religion was another commonality in Kees and Sitje's lives. It seemed to me that religion governed their lives through its fundamental religious laws of the Dutch Reformed Presbyterian Church. My Dad often talked about how he attended church services three times every Sunday when he was just a boy. He would walk a long way with his family to church and a long way back home again, which gave the family just enough time in between trips to energise with food for the next leg of the journey. Dad's mother would prepare the family food on Saturday for Sunday meals and wash the dishes on the Monday so that the family could honour Sunday, the Sabbath a day of rest, dedicated to their worship. Dad told me that he adored his parents. In my mind I felt for him having to live within the strict controls of these unbending laws. Incredulously it seemed to me that my parents and people around them were totally controlled by religion which appeared to feed into the strict social constructs of tradition and culture in their part of the Netherlands during the early 1900's. Mum and Dad told me that in their day religion played a major role in people's lives where people would support and vote for the Netherlands political leaders according to their religious alliances

Kees's parents passed on when he was a very young man. He then became legally responsible for his five younger siblings. Kees was a gentle soul who took his responsibilities seriously. By default he became the legal guardian for his younger sisters and brothers. My Mum said, "Kees was the pick of his siblings to become the family guardian because he was a sensitive man, who cared for people especially his own family."

Mum adoringly told me that in his youth Dad was tall dark and handsome with a mischievous glint in his blue eyes. Though I remember his blue eyes sunken with age, framed with black eyebrows contrasting with his olive skin. Even then towards the end of his life his smile put an infectious glint in his eye, still lighting up his sunken old face. Dad told me that he was bound by law not to marry, until his siblings left home or were old enough to be independent.

My mother Sitje told me that during her five years of courtship with Dad, they were governed by the strict ruling of the Dutch Reformed Presbyterian church which decreed that couples maintain a platonic relationship until they were married in the eyes of the church. If the couples transgressed and especially if it became obvious when the woman was with child, they would be obliged to humbly stand in front of the church congregation, who would be witness to suitable admonishment for their crime against the church. The church provided clarity for its congregation of good versus evil and a seemingly clear spiritual path where if followed the chosen would spend eternity in heaven. Sitje lived within these black and white values of her church which decreed her life's pathway. These values would live with her forever becoming her guiding light to build her own life and that of her children. It seemed to me that her pledge to her religious belief was unwavering, as it was with her mother and her mother before her.

Sitje was an attractive blue eyed fair haired short woman who stood around five foot who was blessed with ageless skin. For a short woman Mum often stood tall. She was the respected matriarch of her family and was driven to have her family respected within her social and religious community.

Sitje had a fierce sense of right and wrong and an equally strong sense of loyalty. She took her wedding vows seriously and obeyed her husband through supporting his decisions and she was there to provide him with strength when needed. It mattered to her what people thought. I perceived that my mum had a strong fear of judgement, as she intimated to me that she felt that her in-laws were constantly very critical of her. Sometimes tears would well in her eyes when she talked about where she fitted or did not fit into her new family. In my mind this criticism was an effective catalyst in her decision to choose to move her whole family to another country. Sitje would step out of her comfort zone to leave behind her country, her culture and everybody she knew to support her husband and provide her family with better life opportunities in a younger country.

All of Kees and Sitje's children would inherit this tenacity to overcome the obstacles in their lives and make the most of what they had, for this I would be very grateful. Kees and Sitje patiently continued their plutonic relationship until they were finally allowed to marry just before the beginning of the Second World War.

Kees was a fine pastry cook and with Sitje ran a shop from the ground floor of their three story mansion. The ovens and bakery were out the back near the stables. It was in this house that Mum and Dad were raising their children, my older sister Sjanie, my big brother Jake followed by my other big brother Matt. The younger of my two brothers was born at the Second World War's end.

Sjanie was Kees and Sitje's little princess, the apple of her parents' eye. She had inherited her mother's beauty. Sjanie had fair hair, blue eyes, perfect teeth, and flawless skin. My Mum would dress Sjanie in quality clothing to show her off. Her aunts would fuss over her. Sjanie would stand patiently while her aunts measured her for her new outfits that they would painstakingly sew for her. Jake was cute with blue eyes and white blonde hair. He was easily entertained. Mum would tell me how Jake would sit in his playpen for hours entertaining himself with the toys he was given. Matt according to mum was her demanding child. If there was mischief to be had Matt enjoyed it and if there wasn't he would make it. Mum said that she needed eyes in the back of her head to care for Matt.

Matt was a loving boy whose face carried expressions of innocence. He was the baby of the family for many years. Unlike me and my brother Matt, Sjanie and Jake endured the German occupation during world war two, sharing their country and their home with the enemy, Hitler's German Soldiers.

During the German occupation hundreds of German anti aircraft guns were located on the banks of the dyke across the road from Kees and Sitje's home. These anti aircraft guns were positioned continuously at the ready, pointing towards the skies.

"When the Germans' fired their guns they would light up the skies like a massive fireworks display. If it wasn't so tragic the light show would have been awesome. The anti aircraft guns fired at unwelcomed airborne vessels unless there were other aircraft in the air to fight for them," explained Kees. My eldest brother Jake told me how he remembered watching planes dog fight through the lounge room window. Even though Jake was only eighteen months old he said that the image remained with him like a slide in his mind.

As the war intensified around my family's home my family were evacuated. To where and for long I am not sure. When they returned to their home they found devastation according to my Mum

"When we returned to our home after the evacuation there was much damage to our home. Valuables were stolen, like my Belgian crocheted bedspread. Food was stolen from the shop." Mum paused, "I couldn't believe that your Dad's letters from me were strewn across the street for everyone to read. I told him to destroy them but no, he had to keep them," She said disappointedly. Her brow furrowed as she continued to tell me her story. "Those letters were private not for everyone to read. I destroyed the letters Kees sent to me. I thought he did the same. He should have done."

The privacy of those letters was clearly more important to my mum than the destruction to their home and business, which was devastating in itself. I pity the perpetrators should they be found. I know that I grew up living in fear of not doing as mum told me too. For a little woman she commanded great respect.

The Second World War was clearly a time when there was more than the physical destruction of war manoeuvres and fighting. I remember listening to stories about how horsemeat was substituted for beef for the civilian population in the Netherlands. War atrocities entered every crevice of people's lives not only threatening their existence but threatening their primary needs and food sources. In Europe soldiers from both sides received food as a priority to strengthen them for fighting. The local population were limited by food coupons. It was a time when people often went hungry from lack of food or lack of ingredients for making good food.

Mum said, "During the war the strong people with a little extra weight covering their bones stood a better chance of survival. The food crisis continued for some time after the war finished." She thought for a bit and then continued to tell me, "If you were fat you were considered to be prosperous"

"People suffered. They would substitute ingredients to replace what they couldn't get. Bread would often be mushy and sometimes runny in consistency and often lacked essential nutrition," Dad added.

Kees and Sitje were a little more fortunate than many and were grateful for their abundance. They would give thanks through prayer before meals and then after meals they would read from the bible, finishing with another prayer of thanks. This practice became a ritual for the rest of their lives. I could see from their photos that they appeared lean in stature. Providing an essential service like food supply through baking and cooking meant that my family had slightly more access to food than the majority of the population even though they were limited through the food coupon system. It was my understanding that the coupons represented the food that came and went from Mum and Dad's bakery and shop, and every other food source.

Like lots of Dutch people living in the Netherlands, Dad's mode of transport was a pushbike. His bike was specially fitted with a large basket attached to the handle bars spanning the front wheel, so that he could deliver his freshly made breads and baked delicacies to the local people. Dad loved talking about Holland's extreme winters where the snow and cold would see him line his wooden clogs with newspaper to keep his feet warm. He needed warm feet to pedal his bike to deliver his artistry to the local population.

I was in awe of Sitje and Kees's courage and heroism during the Second World War. To me they will always be my heroes. They joined the Dutch underground because they were fiercely loyal to their country and its people. They wanted to contribute to the fight against the Nazis. Kees risked his life many times whilst smuggling food to people in need. My Dad told me that, during the German occupation years, he would fill suitcases with food and travel by train to the city to deliver sustenance to people in need.

He said, "I was very lucky that my suitcases were never checked when my travelling permits were checked. I pretended to be a traveller. I must have looked authentic because I was never questioned about the contents of my suitcase."

Towards the end of the war someone had drawn anti Nazism propaganda across Kees's bakery wall. Dad was a bit vague about the messages on his wall and who had written them. He did however tell me that he was carted off for questioning by the Green Gestapo. He was frightened but fortunately for Kees he had a larrikin streak and the Gestapo interrogators gave up on him. He was released after twenty four hours of questioning. The Gestapo believed him to be war crazy. I could understand why one would think that Dad was crazy. He told me secretly about a time at the very end of the German Occupation when he sneaked out at night after Mum fell asleep, to cut the wires that linked the detonators to blow up the sluices just beyond his front door. The Germans wanted to leave Holland's allies with a mess, not clear waterway access to the main rivers in Europe. Kees had risked his life to foil their plans. Dad told me that he was frightened by the evilness of the Gestapo but his fear for living under Hitler's rule was greater. Dad was steadfast in his belief and had the tenacity to fight for what he believed in. The bottom line was that he believed that he and his family were entitled to the best future that was available in this world, with the belief that whilst God was by his side he was able to fight for his choice. Inherently I liked to think that I displayed this same determination when it came to taking responsibility for moving my life forward after tragedy and illness in my life.

On another occasion when Dad was an old man and I was a young woman he told me about a time at the end of the war where a very young German soldier appeared from his hiding spot in the long grass on the dyke wall across the road from Mum and Dad's home. This young soldier shot at my dad as dad cut the wires that were linked to the German's detonator. He said, "This soldier must have only been just sixteen years old. His heavy rifle seemed too big for him. The young soldier pointed his big heavy rifle at me. His rifle seemed to waver in the stillness of the night and then he fired at me. The bullet just missed me. I ran so fast before he could take another shot." Dad's milky eyes stared into the distance as he recalled the enormity of the situation. "The German soldier was so young, so untrained and I believe that's why his shot missed me," Dad's lip quivered. Then a smile crept across his lined saddened face as he told me how grateful he was to have survived, to slide between the sheets of his warm bed without disturbing Mum. "It was better that she didn't know," he said. Dad's smile disappeared, tears pricked his eyes as he continued to share his story with me, "The young German soldier obviously lacked training and appeared to be one of the many that were subscripted to fill the position of real soldiers. Intelligence feedback said that there were many young German boys who were forced to fill the empty boots of the dwindling force of the German Military."

Dad went on to talk about the years during the German occupation of Holland when German soldiers were billeted in his house. His house was large with more than enough room for others to share. Dad said that it was hard living under the same roof with enemy soldiers. Mum talked about one of these billets as a conscripted German soldier and not as an enemy. She said that one particular soldier gave her a bottle of wine for mother's day which she put away until the end of the war. Like Dad she too had a sad face which she covered with pride when she said, "It was good wine but he was still the enemy. I knew its value in times of food scarcity and could not just throw it away. I couldn't drink it or allow any other family members to drink it either."

Mum was staunchly loyal to the Dutch and their allies and the Netherlands people. Even though the German soldier who was living under her roof was a conscript and a decent human being he was still the enemy. A smile crept across her face when she said, "he asked us to his wedding which he was planning for after the war."

Dad would tell stories about when the air raid sirens sounded.

"Mum and I would scoop the children in our arms and rush into the hall way of our house. I would lie over your sister and your mother would lie over your brother until the sirens stopped or the bombs had fallen. We would watch planes fly overhead and the anti aircraft guns fire from the sluices just across the road from our house. The exchange of fire power lit the skies in a myriad of colour." He continued with moisture building in his eyes," The light shows were frightening and magnificent all at the same time." My Dad told me about the day when he heard the sirens. He grabbed my brother Jake from the playpen where he was playing in the front garden and rushed indoors closing the front door. When it was all over Dad said that he opened the front door to an image of destruction.

"A large piece of shrapnel had fallen directly where Jake had been playing. Then I saw an injured young German soldier slumped in the front doorway where he obviously sought shelter from the attack. The young soldier was bleeding profusely. I carried this injured young German soldier to the nearby school which had been set up as a temporary hospital. I left the wounded man in the care of the Germans and went back home to my family." I would listen quietly, in the hope that he would tell me more.

I imagined my Mum at home forging food coupons so that extra food could be provided for the needy without the German's noticing. I thought that my parents were awesome for what they did during the war years.

There were many more heroic deeds. I knew that there were but my Dad wouldn't go into detail. Tears would well in his eyes when he made reference to those neighbouring families who just disappeared. One day he mumbled that he had tried to help them but they were in denial about the threat to their existence. Their disappearance aligned with Hitler's ethnic cleansing for the survival of the master race practices. I would see my Dad fall into despair when he referred to the atrocities of war. He would not elaborate on his work in the underground. I felt privileged to hear Dad's stories. I found that I was filled with sadness for the atrocities that I could only imagine. With tears in his eyes Dad would later emphatically tell me, "I believe the root of all evil is jealousy." Mum and Dad suffered loss during the war.

Kees and Sitje rebuilt their home twice and reconstructed their lives to move forward after the war years. Mum told me how lucky she felt that not one family member died because of the war and how she thanked God every day for saving their immediate and extended families during the carnage of this war. Mum talked about how the effects of war left its mark on many people, changing their relationships with friends, family and the extended community. During and after the war resentment flared towards the nationals who supported the Germans during world war two, especially those who worked as double agents.

Thirty seven years after the Second World War Mum and Dad revisited Holland where Dad met up with a wartime Dutch Nazi supporter, in fact a double agent who was then working in the local post office. Though many years had passed, the memory of deceit was very raw. Dad quivered with anger as he raised his fist and passionately punched the air.

"You traitor, you double agent, you traitor," he screamed. Mum said that Dad's heart was palpitating, his palms sweated and the tears of anger rolled down his cheeks. Mum had to drag him from the post office.

"I can't believe that such a supporter of genocide could be allowed to walk the streets, and work in a government office, being treated like any other Dutch citizen." Dad slumped.

"Where's the justice?" he questioned.

My mum said that he was so overwhelmed with emotions.

The Second World War had clearly left its scars on my Dad.

CHAPTER NINE

Possibility for change came during the early 1950s when opportunity knocked for skilled European workers to immigrate to Canada, South Africa and Australia. Kees and Sitje seized the opportunity and put forward their expression of interest. They needed to move forward and leave behind them a past life of turmoil, where their house and business were bombed twice during the Second World War. They rebuilt twice using their own money as insurance didn't cover their losses. Nor did their church cover or assist with their loss though the church preached that it was against church law to buy insurance.

My mum told me of a malicious rumour monger who had told their Minister that she and Dad had been selling their wares early on a Sunday morning at the local markets. I believe this was in breach of Dutch Reformed Presbyterian religious law as it was breaking the laws of the Sabbath to not work on the Sabbath or cause others to have to work. Working on the Sabbath was disallowed. Without a hearing, the church ruled that Kees and Sitje would not be helped. My understanding of that revelation was enough for me to begin doubting religion even though I went along with my parent's religious ritual because I cared for their feelings. Well I also feared being showered by hellfire and brimstone if I didn't obey.

Middle aged Kees and Sitje were motivated to move to Australia with the possibility to provide their children a better life and future. Australia would be their country of opportunity, a country across the ocean to the other side of the world which would allow them to distance themselves from the reminders of the tragedies of war torn Europe, and their homeland which was so stooped in tradition and stifling in religious etiquette and judgement that there was little room to move. However Kees and Sitje's timing was a little erroneous as they paid for their entire trip and missed the subsidised voyages by one year. Subsequently these highly subsidised voyages would attract even more skilled European immigrants to build and populate this relatively sparsely populated country called Australia.

My Mum was so proud of my Dad. Her eyes sparkled with pride as she told me, "your father was a highly skilled and a well educated European pastry cook." My mum told me that she thought that the biscuits and cakes available in Australia at the time were boring, or at least in the Australian country town where we lived the available biscuits, cakes and pastries were boring compared to my Dad's pastries and artistry. I reckon that my Mother was right because it seemed to me that Continental pastry cooking became popular in Australia many decades after the fifties. Mum sighed,

"In hindsight we would probably have been better off in a city rather than a country town."

Kees had sailed to Australia three months before Sitje to set up a home for his family. He arrived in Australia at the beginning of winter and found refuge in purpose built immigrant accommodation in Mordialloc, a suburb of Melbourne which was by the sea. Even though there was no snow, it was cold with the winds whipping up from the Antarctic. On those very cold nights Kees would innovatively wrap himself in the carpet from the floor to keep warm in the cold corrugated iron clad accommodation. Throughout Kees's time alone in this new country he proved to be very innovative. In order to be ironed and neat in the mornings Kees would neatly lay his trousers under his mattress at night and in the morning they would liken neatly pressed pants with a crisp fold down the centre of the leg.

Kees had fun in the migrant accommodation with other Dutch people he had met on his journey. One morning at breakfast he spooned vegemite onto his bread thinking that it was apple syrup like he ate and enjoyed in his home country. His Dutch mate sighted the pile of topping. He pointed and spluttered. Words rolled from his Dutch mate's mouth,

"Kees, Kees, It's not apple syrup." Kees was too quick as he lifted the bread piled high with the thick black stuff only to find that the vegemite wasn't sweet and it made his eyes water and his tongue sting. He instinctively spat it out as his new friends rolled about laughing. Needless to say Dad was shocked at the taste and he never developed a liking for vegemite or should I say 'the rotten stuff', as he called it. Even so he later became a naturalised Australian.

After the fun and independence of living in immigrant accommodation, he was excited to be travelling to a mid Victorian country town, to work and find a home for his family. It was then time for my mum with my two brothers and my sister to cross the oceans from Holland in the North of Europe to the Southern Hemisphere in Australia. Mum and Dad had both travelled six weeks on the sea to start a new life down under and the new life started was me.

I had chosen to be born into Dutch arrogance which I prefer to call blatant honesty, blatant courage and everything blatant. My courage would be born from this arrogance that was tempered with a little larrikinism controlled by fundamental religious law. This courage would equip me for my life's ride.

Though my birth was not planned, I never the less came into the world to add value to my family's lives. In fact my mother despaired when she found that she was pregnant as she thought her family was already complete. I caused her to feel ill and tired most of the time during her pregnancy with me. The reality of migrating to a new country was exciting but in truth became very daunting or so it seemed to me. Mum was obliged to give birth in a hospital in this new country. Home births were within her comfort zone. My birth was traumatic as thoughts of nurturing yet another child taunted her. Mum already had to face bringing up my siblings in an environment beyond her comfort zone. This new country with its different language, foreign culture and values challenged her beliefs and her truth. This environment was so foreign to her that it threatened her desire to be able to adequately provide, nurture, mentor and guide her children whom she dearly loved and wanted to protect. My mother told me that she was concerned about rebuilding their lives in this new country to regain the position that they held when leaving Holland where they were well respected within their community. In this new country they were unknown.

My dad however was so excited when I was born that when asked what mum had he replied, "A baby."

"Yes but Kees what is it?" He was asked.

"A baby, a baby," he replied excitedly and proudly. My Dad told Matt, who was the usurped baby of the family that he had a little sister. Matt looked back at Dad with wide eyes and said with an urgency in his voice,

"We have to rush to the hospital and tell mum that I have a little sister."

Tradition was strong in religious families like my Mum and Dad's, which influenced my name. Mum wanted to name my older sister Anna but the family wouldn't allow it. Much to my sister's chagrin she was named after our grandmother. Being far away from Holland however allowed Mum the space to call me Anna with the argument that I was named after her younger sister. Nevertheless the judgement and criticism reached far across the miles from Holland back to Australia. Mum would justify her very existence in Australia allaying the rumours that crossed the seas as she wrote to my aunts in the old country. Mum would tell them,

"Yes we go to church on Sundays and we don't work on Sundays, we observe the laws of the Sabbath."

Mum and Dad's family worried that this new country was a den of iniquity with temptation everywhere. When Mum talked to me about our extended family's fear for our eternal lives I would think, these relatives that I have never met probably think that there are no churches in Australia. They probably base their assumption on the pretence that Australia was settled by convicts, perceived criminals deported far away from mother England.

Life for Mum and Dad and their children was really good in this new country. We lived on a farm, a farm with animals. Dad had found himself a well paid pastry cooking job whilst mum busied herself by taking in Dutch immigrant boarders. Even though it was hard work, washing in boiled water heated from fire lit under the copper, the expanse of land between neighbours provided privacy and the space to prepare for a new life. Observing the 'no work on Sundays' rule allowed my parents to continue to observe their day of rest and worship. They made friends through the church who would remain their lifelong friends. Two of these families kindly provided me with kids my age to play with.

Upon my arrival I was quickly accepted as part of the family. Mum would often tell me that, Jake and Matt at the ripe old age of 10 and 8 years of age respectively, became rather resourceful.

"Your two big brothers built you a billy cart with a cabin lined with velvet to cover the spiky ends of the three inch nails that held it together," Mum told me and continued to describe the saga as it happened.

"Please mum can we have the wheels from the new pram. They're exactly what we need to finish the billycart," My brothers pleaded as they looked directly into her eyes.

"No I need them for the pram," answered Mum.

"But the wheels are just what we need," cried my brothers.

My mother told me that my brothers were not willing to give up easily, but she was stronger than they were. My brothers improvised with some mismatched wheels found lying around the farm. I apparently enjoyed my inaugural billy cart ride as it sped down the hill totally out of control. After rolling several times it came to a sudden stop at the foot of a large gum tree. My brothers ran to my rescue and found me inside, unscathed and gurgling loudly as I happily enjoyed the moment with the biggest smile on my face. And that is the story as I remember it being told to me.

I was lucky to be born into a family who lived on a farm in the western district in country Victoria. My mum was home with me and my siblings would come and go to school each week day. My Dad worked as a pastry cook in the local town. His wages were filling the family coffers to build a fruitful foundation for the family's new life in this country of opportunity. In his middle years, Dad became a licensed car driver for the first time in his life, which enabled him to legally drive his first car, which he called the Morris.

Early every morning he would drive the Morris into town, with a pushbike attached to the boot of his car. The bike was insurance in case of rain, which turned the farm's dirt road into mud. During winter, Bluey the old draught horse was often called upon to pull the car out of the mud. He was the most majestic of draught horses highly intelligent and somewhat stubborn. Bluey tired of dragging the car out of the bog and he let Dad know. The last time Bluey was called upon; he waited until Dad was sitting high on his back and then headed towards the middle of the dam. It didn't matter how hard Dad screamed at Bluey, this draught horse wasn't changing direction. Bluey did however stop when he reached the middle of the dam where he stood obstinately with an instinctive knowing that Dad was petrified of water. Being stuck in water on the back of this massively stubborn draught horse was forcing dad to confront his worst fear.

"Well I almost drowned when I was eight years old. During the First World War, I fell into a large underground water tank. I was rescued by a German soldier. I will never forget that experience and how scared I was," Dad told me. Finally Bluey was coaxed out by my brothers who thought it was an hilarious sight. When Dad slid from Bluey's back his clothes were wet and his brow glistened. Was it dam water that one could smell or was it the smell of fear, a fear of being left in the water? That fear of water that my Dad vowed would never leave him?

CHAPTER TEN

Snot and tears ran down my chin. I was crying so hard. My mum had left me in my cot where I would be safe while she was downstairs working in the newly acquired family business. I was only two years old and suddenly felt abandoned where I was left in my cot all alone for hours on end or so it seemed. I was expected to sleep but I wanted to play. I was used to being the centre of attention. This feeling of abandonment would affect my life to the point of feeling badly about leaving a new puppy at home by itself whilst I went to work. I travelled the long distance home at lunchtime just to check it was okay. I would invariably find it entertaining itself, albeit shredding my clothes from the clothesline or sleeping not weeping like I was when I was left. It was not long after that when I discovered through personal growth and self awareness that in other parts of my life the fear of abandonment, would be much more dramatic, affecting my health, my relationships and my self worth.

When I was two years old we had moved to another town closer to Melbourne where Mum and Dad had made a purchase of a café on the Main Street which I believe was an attempt to replicate that which they had left in Holland. It was my Dad's dream. My mum, well her dream quickly dissolved before her eyes. The money saved to purchase a home for her family, in a town where she was beginning to feel that she belonged, was used to buy a shop in a neighbouring unfriendly Victorian country town, where it appeared to be more difficult to blend in. Mum's black and white beliefs led her to support her husband's decision and stand by her man. We were new to town and we were foreigners with a strange culture. In my mind in this town closer to Melbourne we were met with prejudice, misinterpretation and misapprehension. There was no tolerance for differences in this elitist town. These country Australians were unaccepting of foreigners, often calling them new Australians with emphasis on the new. Their tonality was denigrating and downright nasty

"I'm so glad I was born in Australia," I would tell myself, "I'm a real Australian." Though at a very young age I knew I was different and didn't quite fit in.

My Dad was a talented Pastry Cook. I believe that he was way ahead of his time. He worked hard in his bakehouse where he produced mouth watering morsels of artistic food. My mother and her staff supplemented with a meals menu provided for the café's patrons. It seemed that the local bakers in town who provided the bare essentials of bread and sponge cakes felt very threatened. They dropped their prices in an attempt to undermine my Dad's business. My Dad's shop became the most popular of its kind in town. Mum worked the shop with Sjanie beside her to help with her broken English. Sjanie's motivation to speak English really well was spurred by her exacerbation and humiliation felt when she was initially put into a classroom with children three years her junior. The teacher even changed Sjanie's name. Her teacher made no attempt to even try to understand or pronounce the Dutch version of my sister's name. Sjanie's name somehow became June. If the teacher had persevered she would have found that Sjanie's Australian counterpart name was Jane.

Though this new town to me wasn't New Australian friendly, I learned to love the freedom that it offered me. My earliest memories are of living behind my Mum and Dad's shop front business. The back door of our abode opened to a new world in the back lane where I could play unsupervised with the other kids from the back lane. My older brothers also spent time in the back lane where they made Billy Carts which rolled down the hill to the bottom of the lane quicker than my tricycle could carry me. The back lane spooked me at night though with its blackness hiding the boogie men that my brother Matt told me about. One night he walked with me in the darkness and then ran and hid as he taunted, "Careful, the boogie man is going to get you," Then he disappeared into the black of the night. I looked but I couldn't find Matt nor thankfully could I find the boogie man. I remember realising that I was left all alone. Instinctively I ran as fast as my little legs would carry me. My fear became panic as thoughts of abandonment quickly moved through my mind, "Run fast" I told myself, "Faster than he can." I couldn't see the boogie man I just knew I had to run away from him even though it was hard to see anything while the tears streamed from my eyes. I ran into the back of the nearby pub trying to hide from the boogie man when an older girl chased me with a broom yelling loudly, "Go away you horrible little Dutch girl." She scared me more than the boogie man. I took a deep breath, turned and ran home into my Mothers arms "I'm not Dutch am I?" I sobbed inconsolably.

"No you are Australian born", Mum replied warmly, with great pride. I felt so badly about my heritage, well I really wanted to belong to be an Australian that I would only speak English pretending at times not to understand the Dutch that was spoken at home. This practice did however prove advantageous. Especially those times when Mum thought that I had been misbehaving, driving her to speak loudly to me in Dutch. I would run for the stairs leading to our bedrooms with mum chasing close behind. I discovered that if I were to stop suddenly, turn, look down at her innocently and say "I don't know what you are saying." Mum would stop in her tracks and realise that she had been speaking Dutch not English. Translating for mum took a lot of thought and would always slow her speech and lower her tone. This tactic almost always worked to diffuse my mother's wrath where she would shake her head and gesture to me to go downstairs with her. Mum was so busy with her work that she really only had time to chase me when I needed disciplining that is those times that she knew about. I eventually adapted well to my new found freedom. I was three years old going onto four but canny enough to take every opportunity to scarper into the back lane.

The back lane linked the backs of other Main street shops and businesses. When I was three going on seven it was the norm for families to live in the accommodation behind their businesses, providing me with lots of playmates. We played cops and robbers, climbed trees to pick and eat the ripe red blood plums or ride our tricycles up and down the lane. We were rather innovative for three to four year olds. I only had bible stories or peer group tales to guide my imagination. The kids in the lane taught me how to play spies. We had lots of fun spying on the guy who made ezy sauce, in the big corrugated iron shed across the lane. We would peer through the cracks in the building and pretend that we were spies. If he walked towards the space that we were peering through, we would run away like we were being chased by fire. We only ever saw him pack and stack boxes and put lids on bottles until the day he was missing from the shed. We found him in the portable dunny beside the shed. We saw that his pants were around his ankles and noises of fury were flying from his mouth that was scrunched in between his reddened cheeks. He looked like he was going to explode but we knew that we had the advantage. He couldn't move but we did because the smell was overpowering.

Some days we would have tricycle races down the lane. Though one day I was first to reach the bottom and there to my horror was a horse and buggy with an old smelly man sporting long, out of control, facial hair. He needed a bath so badly, dirt was caked on his skin and his clothes were ragged and too big for him. I froze momentarily when a scream erupted from within me. I yelled, "It's a swaggie, it's the boogie man," I was terrified. My two friends and their tricycles had disappeared. I abandoned my tricycle at the bottom of the hill, fleeing on foot in the opposite direction to safety, where my Dad and big brother Jake would save me. I cried uncontrollably, I cried buckets of tears as I fled on foot up the lane. My Dad and big brother Jake heard me from the yard where they were chopping wood for the bakery oven. They came running down the lane to my rescue.

"What's wrong?" They asked. The colour had drained from their faces and their eyes were narrow slits as they looked past the bright sunshine trying to decipher the situation.

"The man down there," I screamed and pointed.

"Did he do anything to you?"

"No he's just there." I felt really confused, *why don't they understand?* They just needed to look at what I could see. Dad and Jake didn't know of Matt's taunts about the boogieman in the blackness of the night. They tried to soothe the fear from me. Jake took me by the hand and walked to the bottom of the lane to collect my tricycle. The man was still there. I hid behind Jake's legs and peered at the man. The man didn't even notice us. He was talking to someone about packets of seeds that he had in his buggy.

This fear of being misunderstood thus misrepresented would grow with me into my adult life. It would undermine my confidence. I would constantly feel that I had to prove my credibility.

Jake was my hero and especially when the boys in the back lane threatened to beat me up. I would puff out my chest and confidently tell them that if they did beat me up then my big brother would beat them up. I forgot to tell Jake this though but I had faith. Jake had after all saved me from the boogie man a few years earlier just like I knew he would. Jake was really cool in those days. I was a five year old girl and he was a cool fifteen year old teenager who could dance like Elvis and he even looked as cool as Elvis. I was so proud to have him as my big brother.

My sister Sjanie was really special too. At times Sjanie would include me in some of her activities. We used to visit her friends farm where we would bottle feed the orphaned lambs. I loved the outdoors and getting in touch with nature.

When I was seven years old Sjanie moved to the city to further her nursing studies where she shared accommodation in Collins Street, Melbourne very close to the Fitzroy gardens. I missed Sjanie and looked forward to visiting her. Sjanie had met a boy whom I was perhaps a little jealous of. One night when the three of us were feeding the possums in the Fitzroy gardens in Melbourne one of them nipped my finger. I cried and I didn't stop until I saw Sjanie's boyfriend's thumb bleed from around his cuticle, where he too had been bitten by the naughty possum.

I remember feeling very special when Sjanie organised special outings for me to accompany her and her friends. I wasn't so keen on her classical music. I was too young then to realise the healing powers of listening to Mozart. I enjoyed being taken to watch live theatre like the '*King and I*', and experience the sound of the Vienna Boys choir live. I always felt very special when I accompanied Sjanie.

Jake taught me how to ride a two wheeler bicycle. He hung onto the back of my bicycle seat as we rode side by side downhill towards the bottom of the lane. At least I thought he was hanging on to the back of my bicycle seat.

"Look you are balancing on your own." Jake said. I remember looking back and realising that Jake had released his connection.

"Oh no you're not holding on to me," I screamed and instantly toppled off the bike.

"You were balancing on your own. I wasn't holding on at all. It just looked like it right at the start. You were doing so well," Jake said, trying to disguise the grin that was creeping across his face.

I sat on the bitumen laneway starring at him. I was really cross with him. Not that I could remain cross with him for too long. I adored my big brother Jake, I thought he was invincible.

"You tricked me. I'll show you that I can do it," I sobbed.

I picked my bike up. Jake steadied my bike holding onto the back of the seat while I got back on. He let go and said," You did ride by yourself, you can ride by yourself again, and I will stay close while you do it." I quickly learned to love the freedom of riding my bike anywhere I wished in this country town. Except for the day when I flew down the back lane just behind Coles and crashed into another bike crossing my path. The other bike hit my front tyre pushing my front wheel which spun side ways. My handle bars cut into me and left a bit of a hole in my side which leaked a little blood. *Nothing that a band aid can't fix,* I thought, but it did hurt. I cried when I showed my mum. She disinfected and covered it with a band aid. A hug and a band aid healed real wounds in those days. These were the days of innocence when I had the confidence and the determination to do whatever it took to overcome the obstacles to achieve my goals. I was safely cocooned in a family of big brothers and a sister who mostly looked out for me. My Mum and Dad were close by but busy working in their business which gave me the freedom to explore my world. I loved the adventure of the back lane and later the freedom to explore further into the town and its surrounds.

My other older brother but younger of the two, Matt was best friends with my best friend's brother Jed who lived next door behind the bank. Then two doors down the lane from our place lived a pawn broker and his family. They were mean people as the pawn broker's wife would chase me down the back lane accusing me of fighting and hurting her son Michael. I think Michael's older sisters lay blame on me for their wrongdoings. Eventually I did fight her son Michael. I was sick of his taunting. His sisters would whisper in his ear telling him that he was to accuse me of being a dirty little immigrant kid. Michael was attacking my self esteem adding to the confidence bashing of other prejudiced people in the town. "I'm not a dirty immigrant. I was born in Australia. Don't you ever call me that again," I screamed loudly for his sisters' benefit. Michael's sisters' whispered in his ear and then Michael hit me. The day I fought Michael he came off worst and it would be my short victory. He was a scrawny little blonde kid. At the time I thought, *His sisters probably stole is food. Well they were fat and he was skinny, that's why I sing to them, fat and skinny went to war and fat got killed by an apple core.* I remember that my thoughts were interrupted when his sisters ran to tell their mother on me. Michael's mother appeared out of nowhere. She was furious and chased me down the back lane, eventually cornering me in the chemist's backyard loo. I had hoped that she would give up the chase but not this time. I could hear her scream, "Where are you, I will find you." I felt like a trapped animal. I looked through the gaps in the door praying that she would turn tail and go home but this prayer wasn't working. I could see under the gap that her big feet were stamping towards me. She wrenched the door open and started hitting me and yelling very loudly, "You beat up my little boy. Don't you dare do that again? Who do you think you are? You're nothing but a dirty little immigrant girl."

She hit me hard. I cowered under my arms trying to protect myself from her big mass but she had made contact. It was then that I truly knew she was mean. I continued to raise my arms protectively in front of me peaking through the open spaces around my skinny arms. I could see steam pouring from her every orifice. Michael's mother, the pawnbroker's wife's eyes were dark almost black, her nostrils flared and her mouth showed lots of yellow teeth as her tonsils danced in the back of her throat. Her little boy was right behind her sniggering at me. Suddenly Michael's mum twisted her gnarled old body towards him. Yes my imagination was in overdrive. She was horrible and that is how I saw her in my mind's eye. Michael instantaneously turned on the tears. She grabbed his arm and stomped up the lane back through the steal bars that protected the back of her house.

The pawnbroker's wife was disliked by the local kids who would inadvertently serve my revenge. Stuff always happened when I was tucked up in bed, but I made it my business to hear about the goings on in the back lane. I carried this interest of local knowledge into my work life. There were times in the workplace where I needed to give new staff the heads up about my local knowledge. Like who was connected to whom and who had the influence of power.

I remember seeing a photo of my Dad leaning against the back wall of his bakery appearing to listen to the two boys who were holding the handlebars of their bikes. The boys appeared to be in deep conversation with my Dad. When I asked Dad about the photo he smiled and told me his story and this is how I remember it.

"Who's out there?" screeched the broken man the pawnbroker through the velvety stillness of the black night. "If I catch you I will kill you," he shouted.

Two doors down the backlane from our café and our home's backdoor was the Pawn Broker's dwelling, fitted with bars like those in the local police station's prison cells. I was only three years old when I first saw these bars and I still recognised them from my Dad and my visits to the police station cells at the top of Main Street on our mission to deliver hot meals for the inmates.

The same types of bars fitted on the pawnbroker's house were an invitation for mischief for some of the older boys who frequented the back lane. They would put their sling shots or rifles to good use, regularly shooting out the street light in the back lane which illuminated the Pawn

Broker's backyard. The boys would then run as far away as possible but stay close enough to see that every time the Pawn Broker would appear red-faced with smoke coming out of his ears. The pawn broker was particularly disturbed after the night where two boys with a bucket of cold dirty water in hand, climbed on the roof of his lean to bathroom. Everyone in the back lane knew that the Pawn broker's family bathed on a Saturday night. Six o'clock every Saturday night the pawnbroker's kids would have to run home in preparation for their Saturday night bath. From the boy's vantage point of leaning over the roof of the pawnbroker's bathroom they could see through the large gap between the tin wall and the lean to roof, left there to allow the bathroom steam to escape. The boys sat on the cold roof warmed by the wafts of steam escaping the Pawn broker's bath water. They could hear the splashes while the Pawn Broker happily wallowed in the warmth of his pleasurable Saturday night bath. The sound of water rising and falling enmasse whilst the large body levered itself out of the water alerted the boys to lean over the edge of the roof and peer through the gap, just in time to see the Pawn Broker get out of his bath, dry himself and put on his pristine, clean white underwear. They smiled at each other, signalling to act quickly. They tipped the bucket then heaved its contents of cold dirty water through the gap. They had accurately aimed the contents at the man clad in his clean set of underwear for the week. The boys watched as the pawnbroker froze when the water hit him. It was like his feet were bolted to the ground. His body swelled as he inhaled deeply. The Pawn Broker's face changed colour to that of a deep red ruby.

"He's going to explode." The boys whispered mischievously.

A roar heightened to its intensity as the Pawn Broker exhaled.

"You bloody kids, I'll kill you," He screamed. The boys watched from the safety of their hiding place where they squatted on the roof, behind the chimney. They stifled laughter as they observed the outcome of their handiwork. The Pawn Broker stood in the light of his back porch. Through the bars, the boys could see that his underwear was a murky muddy mess. He stood soaked with steam rising from his warmed body through the cold film of murk dripping towards the ground below him. He was outraged shaking his fist in the air, whilst stumbling through his angry repertoire. He was peering into the blackness of the night seeing nothing. The street light was out again.

"He'll need to have two baths in one week and another set of clean underwear. That'll teach the cranky old bugger to mess with us," one boy said to the other.

"Teach him to accuse us of shooting out his back light," they told my Dad. My Dad never revealed their identity but the story made him smile. His eyes twinkled with mischief. He looked up at the ceiling and then back to me as he recalled his childhood adventures in Holland. Filled with mischievous laughter he told me about how he and his mate would hide outside a nearby neighbour's outhouse waiting for a particular lady to use the can. In those days the full cans would be removed and replaced with an empty one by the night man. The full can would be removed from under the toilet seat, via a trapdoor at the back of the outhouse. One dark evening Dad and his friends had carefully removed the can from under the toilet seat and waited until the woman was carefully poised on the seat. Hidden in the blackness of the night the boys then quietly lifted the flap of the trapdoor at the back of the dark outhouse. The boys used a straw broom to tickle the woman's bare bottom. The poor woman shrieked, knocked over her candle, and ran from the outhouse building. "She couldn't see a thing in the black of the night," Dad said, smiling broadly.

As a child I would relish the tales of my Dad's childhood in Holland during the early nineteen hundreds. It was like he lived on a different planet.

For relaxation families would warm themselves by the fire whilst they chatted or sat with their needlepoint or read books or discussed the events of the day. It was a time without television, computers and computer games. Generally speaking people were not as well educated in the formal sense of education. It seemed that not many books were published other that the classics or the bible. My Dad drew me a picture of a well disciplined work lifestyle. People power was the resource in the workplace without computers and the technology to work for them as it does for us today.

I got the impression that in my mum and dad's world the discipline that was needed to successfully perform at work flowed through to their social and family life which was governed by religious and political rulings, a conditioning Mum and Dad brought into their own family. However my freedom to play and entertain myself whilst Mum and Dad's time was consumed with running their business allowed me to develop an individual streak. Whilst Mum and Dad were busy I lived by my own unwritten rules. For example I loved to climb trees and the higher the tree the better. If the bottom limb was too far from the ground for me to lift myself into the tree I would find a way to clamber up the trunk to start my climb. I would climb, limb by limb to the top and then down again. The more challenging the tree was to climb the more alluring it was for me.

I didn't have the constant discipline conditioning from a parent who was continuously by my side, structuring my life for me. I knew that I had to be home for meals, home by dark, and go to church and Sunday school on Sundays. Sunday was to be revered as the Sabbath, the holy day where people were meant to worship God, a day of rest. Of course I went to school during the week as well but the rest of the time was mine.

In contrast it seemed to me that my mum and dad had lived a very structured life where they were guided right down to their political voting preferences. I remember my Mum saying, "In Nederland we voted for the political party aligned with the Dutch reformed Presbyterian Church. In Australia we're confused because there doesn't seem to be any religious alignment with political parties, expect for perhaps the Democrats aligning with the Catholics and we're not catholic. We've been brought up to believe that the Catholic religion is not the true religion for us. Who do we vote for in the State and Federal elections?" I watched my mother. I could see worry creases in her face form around her mouth and forehead. Mum would chew the inside of her mouth as she stared into the distance. *This is really serious*, I would think. I had little understanding of governance I just felt that religion and politics caused pain at least on my mother's face they did.

As a special treat for her children, my Mum would regularly read children's bible stories to my sister and brothers on a Sunday afternoon. My brother Matt later told me how he would stare at the door that would open to his freedom willing it to open and take him away from these stories. Matt was an outdoor boy. He later told me that he found the bible stories uninteresting and even depressing at times. He just wanted the freedom waiting for him on the other side of the door. *Mum didn't spend time reading me bible stories,* I thought feeling sorry for myself.

Matt was finally released from Bible stories when Mum and Dad worked in their business during the week and on Saturdays. Drained of energy Mum and Dad would literally rest on Sundays between church services. At times they would share a meal or visit friends after church for coffee. Sometimes we would venture out on a picnic with others from the church. Never would they purposely cause work for themselves or someone else on a Sunday.

Mum and Dad worked hard in their business and there was no conserved energy to further torture Matt with bible stories. Instead we played in the back lane where my brother Matt and his friend Jed made the most of the outdoors. At the tender age of 12 they proved to be quite inventive, especially when they taught me as a four year old how to make a cat sound like a bagpipe. Wanting to please them I picked up this friendly cat in the back lane. I thought carefully about their instruction and proceeded to put the cat's body under my arm, his tail in my mouth and I then pumped his body with my arm as I bit its tail. The cat screamed in between pumps. They were right it did sound like a bagpipe. I was most upset though that the cat kept its distance from me forever more.

Jed was really horrible to animals and especially his dog who was then horrible to me. He had dog called Ether who bit me just because I was standing near its food. Jed's mum heard the screams and came running out with chocolate to soothe my pain. "Are you okay?" she asked. "Here have some chocolate; it will make you feel better." I sobbed and gulped and almost choked eating this delectable delicacy. I was used to meat, vegies, fruit and bread. A chocolate bar as a special treat was kept for Sundays. The dog had bitten me mid week. Besides I didn't feel like eating chocolate. I was probably in shock and not a bit hungry, especially for the sweetness of chocolate. I forced myself to eat the chocolate even though it made me feel sick. I ate it because Jed's mum told me too. I was already trying hard to please people around me.

Every November 5th Guy Fawkes cracker night, Ether would run into Dad's bakery and hide under the benches as close to Dad as he could get. One cracker night early in the dog's life, Jed had experimented with a lit threepenny bunger cracker which he stuffed under a jam tin with the dog seated on top of the tin. When the cracker exploded, it spewed the tin with the dog on top into the air. Jed probably called it the flying dog. And that was the beginning of the dog's life. I don't know that anything horrible happened to Ether after that.

Saturday nights were my treat night with just me and my Dad. We would walk to the top of the main street to the local milk bar where I was allowed to choose an ice-cream. I loved this special time with my Dad.

At the ripe old age of seven I excelled at church attendance where I won an attendance award. I had attended regularly for five years and was presented with a leather bound bible, a grown up's bible for my trouble. I think I was the youngest ever in this church to receive this award. My mum and Dad attended church twice a Sunday every Sunday, so how could I miss? I enjoyed the camaraderie of fellow church children but often thought that the collection money Mum gave me should go toward lolly purchases. I feared hellfire and damnation so I didn't succumb to that temptation. I just watched as my friends filled their faces with lollies bought from the shop across the road with their two shilling pieces. I was amazed that they weren't struck by lightning for making someone work on the Sabbath to serve them the lollies. The thought of punishment befalling them was scary enough to stop me buying the mouth watering delicacies. During the throws of temptations I was rather excited to hear Mum having a conversation with one of the sinner kid's mum who had offered my services in a church play which was about Dutch children.

"Oh yes bring her along, we'll let her know what she has to do and say when she gets here. It will be wonderful to have a real Dutch girl in the cast," The director said. I was too young to notice patronising sarcasm or innuendoes in their conversation. I just felt excited to be included but really nervous because I didn't know what was expected of me, other than I needed to wear the Dutch national dress. Time passed and I hadn't heard from anyone about the play. I was sent along with costume in hand only to be made to feel really small and invisible as everybody ignored me. I waited patiently on the sidelines and tried to imagine what I would be doing on stage. My feelings soared from excitement to fear.

What if they throw me on stage and expect me to adlib or sing solo, I thought in trepidation. Time was running out, the show was close to its start and no-one had spoken with me. Eventually the Director strolled towards me. She said quite sharply, "Anna we don't need you in the play. We already have enough people." I got the message quite strongly that I wasn't needed and that I wouldn't be needed. Even though I was rather relieved, feelings of rejection soared. It was after all my mother's idea. I could blame her. I didn't realise at the time that my mum was trying to make good things happen for me. Most of the time my mother took care of my basic needs but that is all the time she had for me. Mum and Dad both worked long and hard taking time from the family to work in the family business for the family's future. Sunday was set aside for family time or should I say family worship time. Other than Sundays I would basically see my parents at meal times when Dad would sit me on his knee particularly when I refused to eat. He would play aeroplanes with the food on my spoon. I loved the attention and the humour and would eat anything in return. Instead of smuggling my greens into the dogs mouth under my chair or hide whatever food I detested in the room's fireplace.

I was nearly eight when my invisibility nearly ended as Mum and Dad prepared to put their business on the market. The business had grown, it really was successful. Mum and Dad only had to visit the Solicitor to sign the lease for another five years, and then it would be market time.

Sitting in Mr Crook, the Solicitors' Office full of excitement and expectation my Mum and Dad quickly asked where they had to sign. Their dreams were about to be realised. They had built a future for themselves and their family. Their hard work had finally paid off.

"I'm sorry but I have redrawn the document as the shoe shop business across the road needs to relocate and your building is the only potential vacancy." The Solicitor said. His face was devoid of expression as though he were rattling off a list of facts to someone who had no interest.

"This is almost worse than the war, worse than the bombs destroying our house and business. How could anyone steal our business? This is not happening." Was all they could say to each other? "You can't do this." They said to the solicitor in unison.

"I just did." Mr Crook said stony-faced.

Faces ashen and bodies in shock Mum and Dad angrily but sincerely told him, "We will take this to the highest court in the country if we have to." They trudged away not believing what had transpired. The shop was to be dissembled and some of the fittings would be sold on for a paltry amount. I sat and watched as I sensed that my life seemed to destruct before my eyes. I listened and caught bits and pieces of what was happening. I watched the long faces with tears rolling down cheeks towards the floor, where legs passed by me, outstretched arms were pulling fittings off walls, I saw the place that had been my home literally being pulled apart in front of me. I understood that life as I knew it was stolen from me and my family.

My grade three teacher, who always dressed in black or dark navy, crepe dresses, who wore sensible walking shoes and wore her hair just as sensibly with it pulled severely into a bun at the back of her head often glared at me over the rim of her glasses. I believed she hated me, but this day she called me up to her desk to inquire about what was happening to my parents' business. She drew me near with her arm around my waist. I clung to any warmth and care that was dished out to me. I didn't care that this woman dressed in black crepe with her hair bundled on top of her head was just gossip seeking. Not quite understanding, I repeated what I had overheard,

"Mum and Dad had built a business to sell and Mr Crook, the evil solicitor stole it from under them."

She listened and quickly dispensed with me." You can go now. Go sit down at your desk Ann" she said almost gently.

Living in the back lane ended abruptly. I felt abandoned with nowhere solid to place my feet. I didn't understand what was happening but I knew that life as I knew it would never be the same again. Discrimination seemed to soar. I hated deeply as my being filled sadness and anger. I felt helpless with rejection and abandonment filling my soul. I had managed to understand that Mr Crook, the crooked solicitor whom our family trusted had taken away our whole family's future. I later understood that Mr Crook didn't tell my Mum and Dad that he was representing both parties interested in leasing my Dad's business premises. He probably thought that my parents who were heavily accented and new Australians wouldn't understand the issues revolving around conflict of interest. Mr Crook just walked over us and kicked us where it hurt including me. The other party was an Australian with the only shoe shop in town. I heard rumours that the shoe shop building was resumed by the banking company who owned the building. He was kicked out and then he kicked us out. I felt very confused.

Where will mum buy my shoes? I remember thinking,

Dad will probably have to fix them with the sticky stuff he uses to stick new soles over the old.

I was only seven going on eight years old when I experienced this surreal reality where all the grownups were functioning mechanically around me doing what they had to with tears in their eyes. It was like I was an invisible observer. Nobody stopped to tell me what all the sadness around me meant. They probably thought that I was too young to understand. More than likely they were trying to protect me. I had no idea how I was supposed to react. My basic routine remained the same. We still said grace before and after meals. The readings from the bible after every meal became even more sombre. *I hate that man for making my Mum and Dad cry,* I thought over and over There were so many aspects of this experience that carried on to my adult life. What was the point of climbing to the top of the highest tree when I had experienced my family's tough climb to success taken from our control in a heartbeat? These feelings of insecurity and uncertainty would carry over into my adult life. It wasn't until I explored my timeline and realised that my family were actually protecting me and keeping me safe. I discovered that they hadn't realised how much I did understand and how invisible I felt. I would learn much later in life through nlp studies that my defining moments that were formed between the ages of 0-7years of age were where we form beliefs through an unconditional acceptance of modelling our environment. Many of my journey processes have been about different aspects of this experience. My life as I knew it at the age of 7 years was stolen from me, leaving me with the feelings of helplessness, unworthiness, sadness and abandonment.

CHAPTER ELEVEN

We moved into shared accommodation with an elderly gentleman with gout. Mr Wood was a rotund well dressed man who kept pretty much to himself. He couldn't look after the house on his own so it served him to have Mum cook and clean for him and Dad and the boys would do the maintenance around his house. It meant that I would go to another school, a much newer school on the other side of town. I was so excited to live in a real house with a garden and my Mum wasn't working. She was home when I got home from school and I always had afternoon tea waiting for me. I enjoyed having a mother at home and came to expect the same every single day. Until the day I saw a note on the door telling me that Mum was next door. I panicked and read the words on the note taking their meaning literally. I went to the next door of the house but this door was also locked. Every other door into the house was locked too. Fear rushed through me. I was abandoned. I then realised that Mum meant that she was visiting the next door neighbour and that is where I found her.

I loved the evenings in our new home. We would sit around the open fire in the lounge room at night talking or listening to the radio. I always had to go to bed when the conversation started to get interesting though.

Then one morning I woke to an ambulance waiting outside the house. My brother Matt had found Mum lying on the floor in the kitchen. I was quickly given breakfast to eat and sent on my way to school. I remember climbing the hill towards school and stopping to look back to the bottom of the hill below. I could feel a queasiness rise in my stomach. The scene below was surreal. I hoped no one saw the ambulance because what would they think of me. Somehow I thought that I was to blame. I felt bad because I had told my mum that my friend's Catholic Bible was much more interesting than the big brown protestant bible that we had.

"They have a picture of Jesus and his eyes follow you around the room. Our bible doesn't have any pictures like that." I said as I watched my mum's blood boil. It didn't please her that I enjoyed catholic bibles. I hurried to school to put distance between me and the scene behind me. Later that day I realised how real this scene was when I was collected from school by the Reverend from our church. My life in the back lane had been taken from me and now my mother was taken from me. Life swirled around me and before I knew it, I went from staying with the Reverend and his family to a family friend's home.

My family was distracted with worry. Mum had been transferred by ambulance to a Melbourne hospital three hours drive from home. Just as well we had friends with whom our family could stay with in Melbourne. I had grasped that Mum was very ill, in fact that she had teetered between life and death. I didn't quite understand the enormity of it all as I remember asking my sister, "Can you plait my hair please Sjanie? I need to look nice when I see Mum." Mum was lying very still in her hospital bed.

"I'm not allowed to move," Mum told us, "They put dye into my throat. It missed and went into the tissue. It felt like tons of bricks were falling on my head, in fact it felt like the hospital walls had caved in and all of them were falling on my head." Mum's face scrunched a little like she was feeling the pain all over again. *Wow* I thought; *imagine the bricks from this building sitting on your head.* I later heard someone say that Mum had a brain haemorrhage. Through some miracle the bleeding stopped.

Mum, Matt and I returned to the country town that we called home. Mum could no longer cook and clean for Mr Wood. We were forced to move to squalid quarters, where we paid less rent. I didn't really mind because we didn't have to live in the same house with the grumpy old man with gout.

I was beginning to understand death though it was a concept that I hadn't needed to consider before my mum was sick. I then found a dead bird in the yard of this dark falling down house that would be our new home. I buried it with the ritual that it deserved. My life had changed dramatically with the back lane gone, my mum was sick and the house we lived in wasn't much better. When I reflect I realise that when I buried the bird I was burying my life as I had known it. Not only was I a new Australian but I was now a poor new Australian. Poverty was new to me and my family and none of us really knew how to deal with it. There were no rule books for this experience. We used to feel sorry for people living the same lives that we found ourselves in and now it was our life. My mum turned to her bible trying very hard to inflict its messages onto me. I had no time to listen to words that made no sense. *Just read the words so I can go outside and play,* I would mumble to myself after every meal. If mum heard my mumblings she would deliberately make me sit longer and listen to more words. I didn't understand at the time but the bible and her religious ways were the only thread left of her previous life.

A few days after the bird's burial my curiosity got the better of me, I wanted to know what happened to it while buried six feet under well six inches under the earth. I had often heard the words death linked with eternity in heaven or hell with its fire and brimstone. I wanted to know what really happens. I wanted to know what happened to the bird. *There's got to be more to death than just a bunch of old dead bones,* I thought. I redug the hole much larger than the original but there was nothing. It truly had turned to dust. I later learned that Mum had dug it up. She didn't want me fiddling with dead stuff.

I was in grade five and nine years old. Life was becoming difficult. Dad was working long hours but not earning enough to support his family in the way he believed they deserved. Dad looked towards the city of Melbourne for better job opportunities.

CHAPTER TWELVE

Jake and Sjanie were already working in Melbourne. Dad stayed with them and they all looked for more substantial work for Dad and a place to live for the family. The duplex house we were to rent was in Hawthorn, an inner middle class suburb of Melbourne. In hindsight it was well located with access to a local library, schools, public transport and shops. Even though the house had a small back and front yard I yearned for the wide open spaces and freedom of country life. People were different here, their lives were more structured. In my mind I noticed a lack of spirit, an absence of seeking adventure, every breath you took was governed by rules and judgements or so it seemed to me. Everything in my world was instantaneously turned upside down. Something as simple as riding a bike was fraught with danger. My mother said, "You might be hit by a car on the busy roads out there." In fact my bike was taken from me. I didn't feel comfortable to walk the streets alone or swim in the local swimming pool by myself. There were too many people in the streets and in the pool. Recreational time for my friends was organised it seemed with ballet or tap-dancing classes even sport. I watched my friends participate in so many organised extra curricula activities. Where I came from we were free to organise our own fun.

I finally joined Girl Guides. At least they went camping and enjoyed a bit of adventure. We would walk along the beach during the cold of winter enjoying the freedom of the open space. We justified our beach walking jaunts with accessing fresh air giving us healing properties from the ocean's waters. Our guide leader didn't agree that it was badge worthy though. Year round we would mix bushwalking, camping and learning to cook over an open fire. It resembled a little of my free life that I had left behind in the country. This changed when I was forced to change guide companies to a group who lacked motivation. What was the point of just attending meetings in the guide hall and doing nothing else? I was bored so I left.

Our family home had moved again. Our Hawthorn house was sold so we moved from Hawthorn to Camberwell where we rented a much larger two story family dwelling. The house was moist to the point where a ceiling fell in on Matt and me whilst we were watching television. Matt was my knight in shining armour though. He grabbed my arm and yelled," Quick get out of here." My legs automatically ran, following Matt who was still tugging my arm. Outside the door we turned to see a white mist chasing after us followed within a split second by a loud bang as the ceiling met the floor. Our sibling relationship had turned the corner Matt was now my hero.

Matt wasn't home very often. He spent most of his time at University or studying at mates' places. I really missed him.

I was entering year nine and the girls' school I attended was becoming very boring with its silly strictness so constricting that one had to ask permission to breathe metaphorically speaking. We were being conditioned to believe that boys were evil with bad intentions. Strict school discipline and religious discipline worked together to dampen my desire to achieve. My life was so structured that the challenges disappeared. I wasn't allowed to be free anymore. Talking to boys was not allowed in fact it was disapproved of. Boys had always been my friends even when challenged with a fight. Though there was a shift in interest happening. I sometimes dreamt of a boy's touch and being cared for as a special friend. Through experience boys were my peers, then I was brainwashed in a strict girls' school to believe that boys were evil and threatening. Through conditioning I lost the ability to effectively communicate with the opposite sex. I put men on a pedestal, initially behaving subserviently in my relationships. Though I have to say I have never ironed my man's underwear nor, in the depths of Melbourne's winter cold, warmed his undies by placing them over a heating duct whilst he showered.

We moved to the city when I was ten years old. I found myself surrounded by crowds of people and lots of cars. It was busy in the city but life itself was so confusing. The kids at school had their friendship groups and didn't allow me in. I watched as others succeeded in areas where I believed that I could have too, but lack of money, lack of parental support because of beliefs stopped me. I had loved athletics, swimming and playing netball. My almost successes were curtailed because they often entailed Sunday sport and that wasn't accepted in the religious parameters suffocating my life. My friend had her athletic coaching on a Sunday. Netball training was scheduled for Sunday morning training. "Can you imagine me missing church to go to training?" I mumbled to myself angrily." What's the point of even trying? It was easier to become complacent and find other ways of entertaining myself.

The swimming pools in the city brimmed with people. I vaguely remember being jumped on from above as I swam in the deep end of a public swimming pool. I was virtually pushed into the area under the high diving board as the pool filled with people. I felt a thud as a body and arms and legs pushed me under the water. My head ached as I was pulled from the pool. I was breathing and life continued. No one seemed to care. I was all alone in this crowd of people. I spent time alone in the country but I never felt as lonely as I did in this crowd. This feeling of loneliness grew with me as I grew without me even realising.

Invasive poverty penetrated further into my life. My mum couldn't afford to go to the dentist. She had her teeth pulled at the dental hospital and was left toothless for some time before her dentures arrived. Mum came to my school without her teeth once because I had forgotten my lunch." Is that your grandmother?" the kids in the playground asked. "No, she's my mother," I said feeling very embarrassed.

My mum's priorities were different to mine. She never lost her religious drive. She was excited to have found a church that was known to the family back in Holland. For me it was tougher than just going to church twice a Sunday. It was so rigid, preaching hell fire and damnation that I trained my mind to drift, building stories which were intermittently interrupted by the minister's voice repeating the names like Calvin. This name was imprinted in my mind for what, I don't know. My mind would wander to thoughts of how I could break into the friendship cliques at school. I would sit still with my hands clasped together in my lap, balancing my hat on my head, wearing my Sunday best clothes, pretending to look at the Minister in front of me who was preaching from the pulpit. I would grasp at the only freedom I could steal; I would allow my mind to wander. *How could I impress Mel to become my friend? Maybe if I were to be carted off in an ambulance after some dramatic scene where I really hurt myself she would be in awe of my bravery, feel sorry for me and want to become my friend.* There were only so many stories that I could build in my mind before boredom set in.

Suddenly I was 14 years old and still in church. I had trained my mind to wander successfully so that when it mattered in the school classroom it wouldn't focus instead my mind would draw me to outside the window of the classroom like it did when I was in church. My thoughts in the classroom would attach to feelings of excitement anticipating the weekend to come. I began to use my mind to plan. I was too young to go to discos. Though my youth didn't stop me from sneaking out to a Saturday afternoon city dance with a school acquaintance, Rita. She was a new Australian too. Rita had emigrated from Scandinavia to Australia with her family. The Saturday afternoon dance that she took me too was tucked away in a back lane in Melbourne. The space was dark and sleazy. Even though it smacked of adventure it also scared me. My new friend had a familiarity with the place saying hello to every second male we saw. I didn't stay very long and left on my own. I discovered much later that Rita was deported back to her home country because she regularly went to this Saturday disco. I never did find out what she got up to. I was glad it wasn't me. Mum's stories of Holland described a much more rigid way of life. Life was strict enough for me in this part of the world.

Shortly after we moved from the spacious damp cement house in Camberwell we moved into high rise Government commission housing flats in South Yarra, which housed 144 families in each block. Even though we lived on the sixth floor of our building the views were of other high density populated buildings. We had moved even closer to the City in a densely populated high density accommodation part of South Yarra. My environment had changed again.

How many people can be squeezed into one city block? I feel like I am living in an ant colony, I thought. It meant that I now had a long way to travel to school. In fact, I could either catch a tram and train or two trains. I would endure yet another difference. My school uniform was extremely conservative with a hemline down to the knees when mini skirts were the go and I had to wear gloves and a hat. The other kids on my block wore their school uniforms very casually. I felt foolish and undermined as a person in my school uniform.

It seemed to me that I was the only one in this urban density who had to adhere to a strict uniform code of blazer, gloves, hat socks or stockings and polished black leather shoes. Our dresses had to be knee length whilst every other teenager from other local schools wore uniforms just covering their nickers. The school was governed by fear, who we called Black Mac as she always wore her black graduation gown with her arms held by her side and both fists clenched. Black Mac was small of stature and short in height nevertheless she was a little being with a commanding almighty presence. She had short black hair framing her face which seemed to stick to her head with curls kicking up at the back of her neck. Her eyes were dark and her top lip was shaded. At school assemblies Black Mac would stand with her shoulders pulled back, her short arms pointed to the ground beside her with clenched fists and a tightly pulled expression around her lips and eyes. She always positioned herself on the top step facing her 800 students assembled in the quadrangle below. This was the only time I appreciated blending with everyone around me who were wearing identical uniforms. Black Mac may smell my fear but would have trouble isolating it amongst this sea of uniforms. This fear would sit with me for many years expanding from this one little person to nearly all teachers.

Black Mac gladly acknowledged her self gratification as she wielded her strength over us scarring us for life. "You girls are to be commended for obeying the school's dress code. One of our ex students from the beginning of the 1900's has said that you look like you have just stepped out of Vogue". *Yeh right only a senile person would think that we were vogue material,* I thought. "Any of you wishing to break the dress code with even a button undone will face a week's after school detention," She yelled into the assembled mass in the quadrangle. At assembly in the main Quadrangle we would all stand quietly in rows according to our year level not game to take our eyes off her. Black Mac was true to her word. My friends and I often wondered if Black Mac were truly human. We knew that she wasn't superhuman because she didn't save us from the horrors in the outside world. It was like she actioned the evils of men upon us.

Travelling a long distance to school by train was at times educational and rather entertaining, though not necessarily in the positive sense. There was a time whilst minding my own business sitting in a crowded carriage where my gaze exposed me to the sight of a much older man dressed in a suit showing me parts of his male anatomy that I had never seen before. Strategically sitting on the seat opposite me, the man carefully placed his newspaper on an angle, exposing himself to me alone. The zip on his fly was undone and pulled to the side. I was instantly curious to see that the skin which was pulled tight resembled plucked chicken skin and then I realised that I should be shocked. I must have looked very conservative and young in my boring blue long school uniform which resembled a woollen blanket designed to cover my female form.

Black Mac had impressed upon us her dislike for men and their intentions. She was protecting her girls or so she seemed to think. *She must not have travelled on the same trains that I do,* I smiled to myself. I imagined her horror at what I saw. On the trains I seemed to attract the flashers and their dishonourable behaviour. At times I sensed danger especially in the deserted underpasses that linked the train platforms up above. I would run as fast as my legs would carry me up the stairs and onto the platform where there were at least platform staff to protect me. Just as well I was a fast runner.

One cold, wintry, wet, typical Melbourne morning I waited patiently on the platform for the old red rattler to pull into the station. It finally came to a standstill and I pulled open the door to a sight I only expected to see on cartoons. I almost felt sorry for a younger man who had obviously exposed himself to an older female who was furiously beating him across the head with her umbrella. "Don't you dare think that you can get away with that again," she raged. They virtually fell out of the carriage together. He was trying to run away from the woman with his hands cupped above his head to protect himself against the umbrella onslaught. She was lashing out at him for trying to humiliate her. Her rage was winning. I quickly moved and chose to get in the next carriage. I sat away from others in the carriage and hid under my felt hat laughing to myself. *That will teach him,* I thought.

Eventually I found a travelling companion, a friend from school, Kylie who had also moved to my part of town. Kylie was an attractive short, blonde, blue-eyed feisty young lady. She always managed to secure the lead parts in the school plays. Entertaining was second nature to her. We were now two strong the next time a dirty old man decided to expose himself. We only experienced a few more times where a man strategically exposed himself to us in our conservative school uniforms with hats and gloves and blazers buttoned so precisely. Kylie would look at him then instantaneously signal for me to giggle loudly. It worked every time. These men would leave the carriage on the next stop feeling rather embarrassed and discouraged.

We spent a lot of time on the train just watching passengers sit like stone statues as they stared in front. Their only movement was with the momentum of the train. It was deadly boring watching people sit silently with bored expressions on their faces, just like sad robots. We decided that we needed to do some creative entertaining of our own. The games began with our loud conversation penetrating the deathly stares of the passengers. The train carriages were packed to maximum capacity on our home trips so we had a fair audience.

With a serious expression Kylie said, "My uncle died last weekend."

"That's awful, what happened." I enquired compassionately and straight faced.

"Well my uncle was playing golf and didn't see the man next to him hit the ball. My Uncle was standing a little too close and the ball flew into his ear through his empty head and out through the other ear. It hit a nearby tree leaving yellow wax marks on the bark and ricocheted back through his nose and out through his mouth. There was blood, saliva and the remnants from the previous meal everywhere. When he stumbled he slipped on his slimy blood and fell hitting his head on a rock which killed him instantly. But not to worry as he will probably be reincarnated as a red golf buggy with carrot coloured stripes" She said quite seriously.

Our audience, the other people in the carriage who usually sat still whilst silently focusing in front, sometimes swaying side ways or up and down according to the sway of the train were aghast. Their eyes were wide and their mouths agape. Some of the passengers even lost the colour from their faces or just turned green. We timed our stories well, alighting from the train, leaving the passengers to digest the information received.

We varied our trips and mode of transport. Sometimes we included a short bus trip. We were quick to grab empty seats. One day a young working girl not much older than we were, challenged us to stand and give her a seat. After all we were in school uniform and she was a working girl. We ignored her but used our peripheral vision to watch her contort he face, narrow her lips and squint her eyes. She continued to stare at us as we alighted from the bus. We stepped off the bus onto the pavement and turned to the young woman and said," well would you have given up your seat if you were three months pregnant?" The girl went red with embarrassment and then white with disgust. These were the days when one didn't talk about such things as pregnancy, because only tarts and loose women got pregnant so young. Single pregnant young women were scorned by society and sent away interstate or were hidden in houses so that the world would never find out about their transgressions. Often the babies would be taken from these girls at birth and given away for adoption. If nobody knew about the pregnancy or the birth then their reputation would remain intact. In my world I remember that there were some girls who would disappear for health reasons and not be heard of again. I was later told about the illegal abortions that some of these girls submitted to, to keep their reputations. Sadly I knew of one girl who lost her life to backyard abortion.

The do-gooders of the time took great delight in telling the world that some of these sullied girls living in the flats near where I lived were caught breaking the law and consequently sent to Juvenile reformatories.

The do-gooders were relentless in their judgement of these girls, who they deemed to be bad. They would say to me and my friends, "If you associate with them then you will turn bad too."

I did meet some of these girls and I couldn't see the difference. One of these girls defied others judgement and decided to keep her baby. I felt sorry for her because she wasn't sure which identical twin was the father as she had sex with them in succession. I guess two dads' are better than one. Judgement was well entrenched in my life. The fear of being judged in the negative would stay with me for many years to come, impacting on life decisions just because of what people would think. I was losing the freedom to play the game of climbing trees. It suddenly became important to those judging me that I meet a nice boy. It was kind of like an unspoken social rule, to find a nice boy to marry. Whatever finding a nice boy meant. I was in the process of being conditioned to think they were all bad. How many times had I heard the comments like, even in this cement jungle there were those nasty boys who were causing pregnancy and the birth of unwanted children. In the face of all this confusing judgement I would try to hang with nice girls and meet a nice boy.

I met Alan at the local football club's Saturday night dance. He seemed really nice to me. He played for Prahran in the under nineteens VFA competition. Although a couple of years older than me I was attracted to Alan immediately. He was handsome, attentive with a warm smile and looked good in those bottom hugging competition shorts that the VFL players wore. I willed him to be my knight in shining armour.

There was much for Mum to approve of. Alan had a decent job in the bank.

He had a private school education and he was a regular church goer.

Alan had three brothers and three sisters. He was part of a large family albeit a Catholic family. I didn't need to tell Mum everything.

CHAPTER THIRTEEN

My dream of my knight in shining armour taking me away to a better life was threatened. The Government was taking Alan from me. He was called up for National Service. The Vietnam War was well under way and Australia was committed to sending troops in to fight along side the Americans. It was law that twenty year old boys were chosen by ballot to join the army. The 'call up' boys were not even old enough to vote. It would be one year later that the voting age would be dropped to eighteen years of age. These young men had no say though some tried to strongly object through conscientious objections, which almost always landed them in Prison for their trouble.

The Vietnam War was controversial, singing artists were even writing songs objecting to the Vietnam War. Groups of university students regularly protested en masse on university campuses. I objected to my man being taken from me. My school friend Kylie and I travelled from school on the train past our usual stop into the City to join a moratorium march through the centre of Melbourne. We wanted to register our objection to National Service and the war in Vietnam. I remembered atrocious stories of the Second World War where people were dragged from their homes, sent to prisoner of war camps, never to be seen again. Kylie and I made quite a statement clad in our very conservative school uniforms. Just as well there were lots of people or we may have been expelled from school again, had we been caught.

I was amazed however at how quickly the attitudes of these conscripted young men changed after six weeks of basic training. I attended the march out from Alan's basic training, just to steal some time with Alan before he was shipped to his next block of training to New South Wales. There was an excitement in the air amongst the boys of prospects to come instead of fear and dread of horrors to anticipate. My protests to the war had in turn become blasphemous instead of supportive. During this phase of objection I had my photo taken holding a placard saying 'no to conscription'? This photo would appear in my school year book embedded on paper for posterity. It was my way of supporting the cause but it had quickly turned to be the opposite. I was hurting. Did I have no control over my life? Was my whole life controlled beyond me? My back lane was taken from me, my mother was nearly taken from me, my country life was taken from me and now there was an attempt to take my nice boy from me. I would not give up without a fight.

I missed Alan so much that I wrote letters to him each day. He was constantly in my thoughts. The contents of the letters consisted of a lot of dribble but I felt it kept him near. The letters were for Alan's eyes only. Like my mother I wasn't happy to find that Alan's older brother found some of my letters and he actually read them,

"Boy were they stupid letters," He said as he shook his head and grinned from one side of his face to the other, "but I got a laugh from them." *How truly humiliated do I feel?* I thought at the time.

Alan and I saw each other when he had leave. Our relationship deepened and we became close. So close in fact that we found a way to marry even though we were under 21. In those days we were under age and had to seek permission from the olds to marry. I couldn't quite come at living together. I couldn't face the judgement of such an unacceptable practice of the time. I wanted to be with Alan and I was trying so hard to go with the rules.

What would people think? I thought. I couldn't take the judgement which would lead to rejection, *living together is considered to be living in sin which contravenes both religions beliefs. My Mum and Dad are fundamental*

Protestants and his Mum and Dad are strict Catholic. Thank Goodness neither were Irish, I thought.

There was enough trouble in Northern Ireland at the time where the Protestants and Catholics could not find common ground. Instead they shot each others knee caps and performed other such atrocities in the name of religious differences, well that was my understanding.

I was nineteen years old, married and free from the disciplines of home, school and church. My husband Alan had been conscripted into National Service and posted to Brisbane Queensland, many miles away from home. Not only was I free but I was married to my soul mate my knight in shining armour. He had rescued me from the depths of my Melbourne life to live a much more relaxed life in God's own country in Queensland. I was happy to follow this man of my dreams. I don't know whether it was his caring blue eyes or his larrikinism, or his sense of humour, or that he saved me, delivering me to freedom.

Our new home was half an old Queenslander house, which was set on top of a hill in the inner Brisbane suburb of Red Hill. In my new home I soaked in the feelings of bliss which emanated from my new found independence. It was great until that night when I had planned to have a quick meal of baked beans on toast. Alan's army friend Joe had planned to join us for dinner. The cupboards were barely stocked anyway as I was limited by what I could carry. I had to walk up and down hills to the nearest shop and carry bags of groceries home with me. I hadn't yet got my drivers' licence but then we didn't have a car either.

In the kitchen I was crouching down to open the lower cupboard below the sink to retrieve a can of baked beans. I reached up and put the can on the sink. The muscles in my thighs began to hurt. I fell onto both knees and crawled along the floor to the cupboard that held the pots and pans. It was bare. I placed both hands on the top of the cupboard to steady myself as I slowly rose to my feet. Half way up my eyes gleaned the dishes piled high.

"Oh my gosh," I yelled loudly to the empty kitchen. "I haven't a clean saucepan or plate" Scanning my surrounds I discovered that my kitchen's total culinary implements were clogging up the sink and the adjoining bench top. They were waiting for someone to wash them.

"I miss my Mum," I muttered loudly to no one in particular. I suddenly realised that I had inherited all responsibility for the domestic chores.

My first paid job in Queensland was in retail and ideally based in the middle of the City's shopping precinct. I was rising in this world's social status. From part time shop assistant in a big variety store, I had risen to being officially employed fulltime in an exclusive dress shop.

During my first week I got a nasty bout of cystitis. I asked one of the other staff, Hilary, to tell me where the nearest Doctor's surgery was. I really needed to go, to the doctor. Hilary knew that there was something wrong because I would leave the floor regularly to race upstairs to the loo. It was quickly fixed with a prescription for antibiotics from the nearest doctor's surgery.

I was beginning my second week as an assistant in this exclusive clothing boutique, in the centre of the Brisbane City's shopping precinct, when the owner of the shop organised a meeting with me. "You have lied to me," she insisted accusingly. She glared at me, her slim body bent across the table, to get closer to me. *All she needed was a bright light to shine on me,* my thoughts were interrupted when the Gestapo like woman continued," I am pleased with your work but I wanted someone to work in this position for a lengthy period. You didn't tell me that you were pregnant. Hilary sussed the information for me. "I felt humiliated. *This condemnation shouldn't be happening here in my new found freedom,* I thought, *I left all this behind me.*

I could feel angry feelings begin to build in my body, "This is no time to be soft," I mumbled very quietly to myself.

I turned and looked her in the eye and said, "In my interview you told me that I had two weeks to decide whether I liked working here or whether you liked me working here."

"Yes" she responded.

"Well I'm not pregnant," Her face changed and a smile almost broke across her craggy face. I quickly continued my repertoire, "and I have decided that under the circumstances I don't like working for you. I'll finish at the end of the week." Well that wiped the smile from her face. I stood up from the table, turned and proceeded to descend the stairs into the shop. I finished my first fulltime retail job after two weeks at the age of nineteen, earning nineteen dollars per week.

CHAPTER FOURTEEN

In the early nineteen seventies the government began withdrawing Australian troops from Vietnam and the conscripted servicemen's time was reduced, they were only required to serve eighteen months instead of two years. The following election saw a major change in Australian Politics as the Labour Party won the election in 1972 and ceased compulsory enlistment for National Service in Australia.

I was so excited to be returning to Melbourne where Alan was to be discharged from his stint in National Service. He rejoined the bank, and we found a flat to rent in East St Kilda in inner Melbourne, close to where we lived when we met. That honeymoon gloss, though, had fallen from our marriage, never to be returned. It was like the Army had changed Alan, but perhaps it was me who had changed. I searched for work and found a library job to apply for, with a special management library located in Kingsway in Melbourne not to far from the Central Business District. Alan had been a little bemused and told me not to waste my time searching for library work,

"Don't waste your time. Just apply for a shop assistant position," He said. He knew I didn't want that. I don't think he realised the pain of humiliation that I had escaped from in my short-lived retail position in Brisbane. Besides I'll show him that I can get a job that appeals to me.

Well I'm more determined than ever to get this job now. I thought to myself. Finally I received a letter advising me of the interview time and place. I just needed to catch a tram and leave enough time to walk a short distance to the library. My outfit was easy to choose as I had only one good dress. It was very short as the fashion of the day dictated but that was okay, because with the invention of pantyhose no one would see suspender belts at the top of my thighs which would have met the hem of my dress. It was my lovely light green crepe dress with embroidery on the bodice. I had bought it a few years before with my Saturday morning earnings way before we were married. My shoes were platform sling backs with moderately high cork heels.

I am determined to get this job. I will show him that I can. I am going to strut my stuff. Oh I can feel those butterflies having fun in my stomach, I thought to myself

The interview began. I smiled a lot and only spoke when I was spoken too. The rest was a blur. I remembered travelling home again by tram. It was peak hour. The tram was full, though I found a seat under the outstretched arm which joined the smelly armpit pointing at my face and God gave me this wonderful sense of smell. *Wonder what he ate for tea last night? Maybe garlic and onion,* I thought to myself.

We didn't have a phone in the flat so I waited for the letter box to give me the good news.

"Yes, I have the job," I bragged to Alan. Of course he was very happy for me. I began my new job and enjoyed what I was doing. Not long after I started the Institute decided to move into their purpose built building in St Kilda, right in the middle of Melbourne's version of the red light area. I never saw any ladies of the night though. It was about a half hour brisk walk from work to my Mum and Dad's where Alan would pick me up every evening to drive me home. I enjoyed my walk. I wandered down asphalt paths, lined with Victorian houses, skirted with tiny lawns and gardens. Several house yards had concrete painted green to resemble grass. There was a particular corner house that I loved with its beautiful renovation of fresh white paint, large sparkling clean windows looking out at the world and a lovely garden with flowering perennials skirting the manicured lawns. It was in this garden that I was often greeted by the ugly bullterrier who stared at me through the fence, interrupting his enjoyment of sunbaking on his back behind the whitewashed slatted fence. He always wagged his tail when he saw me though.

My walks were rarely interrupted. It was a good time for my space. One afternoon a car with a Western Australian number plate slowed and stopped. The driver got out of his car and asked me for directions, "Could you please tell me where Robe Street is?" he asked politely. I was mind reading and very quickly concluded that he was lost and needed direction. I helpfully pointed to the crossroad ahead, "That's it over there," I told him. He hesitated and raised his hand to his head to scratch behind his ear as he said,

"Thank you. Would you like a job love?"

I smiled and politely said, "No thank you I already have a job." I proceeded to walk away from him when suddenly I realised what he meant by a job. Well my heart raced, I instantaneously turned bright red from head to foot like a stop light and walked as fast as I could to get away from him. I felt so embarrassed. *Fancy being judged as a prostitute,* I thought. *That's bad, bad things happen to prostitutes, that's what I'm told,* I thought before almost breaking into a run.

"I didn't realise what he was propositioning me for. Oh gee oh gee! How humiliating," I said quietly to myself. *That will teach me for trying to mind read,* I thought.

The early 1970's saw house prices boom in Melbourne. Alan and I bought our first comparatively young three bedroom house in the outer suburbs of Melbourne for $19,000. It seemed to me that the outer suburbs were attracting young people, well some that I knew, as they renovated their inner city dwellings to sell and raise the money to buy their plots of land further out to build their dream homes.

We only had one car so every morning Alan would drive me to work first and then drive to his work. On my days off I was imprisoned in the house in the outer suburbs unless friends popped around with their cars to take me places. I had attracted someone from a different background who much to my confusion believed, that women were to be kept barefoot and pregnant. Though Alan was happy to embrace women's liberation and have me work to contribute to the family coffers. At times I felt that the caring wasn't there. It seemed that football and the races and his friends were far more important than me. My role was to have dinner on the table waiting for him on his return from wherever he went.

Alan went out a lot without me as my responsibility was domestic and his responsibility was to spend time with his friends, going to the football or the races or just being a boy. Public transport was negligible out there in the sticks. I became rather frustrated and often felt abandoned and unappreciated. My emotional layers were building once again.

Spending time with the person you loved wasn't meant to be like this,' I thought, *I really thought it would be about sharing and having fun.* It got so bad that I talked about my misery with an older woman at work.

"Just leave him," she said. I thought about it but felt somewhere deep down that there was something worth saving. I needed to chill out and understand our differences and work towards harmony. That's when our life started to come together. We were going to have a holiday together.

At work I had often gone out of my way to work split shifts and offered to fill the more unpopular shifts saving the branch librarian's bacon. I wasn't impressed when my request for leave was declined. I needed to spend time with Alan to nurture the upswing of our relationship. So I got another job, just like that.

I had not long changed my job from a special library and I was now changing from a public library to a college library where I was allowed to take some holidays with Alan. As it happened during school holidays one week's paid leave was granted to employees of the college library staff on top of their annual leave. I even got study leave to finish my library technicians' course. I loved my new job and even made new friends. I quickly felt like I belonged.

Alan and I started planning for the future. We sold our first home for a large profit almost doubling our money in two years, which allowed us to move into a larger home closer to the city. We had also started researching the acquisition of land on the south coast of Victoria as a possible future investment prospect. The Bank for whom Alan worked offered one year contracts for staff to transfer from Victoria to their London branch. We would plan for the future to spend a year living in London and touring Europe on holidays.

Our holiday happened and we actioned our first plan for a road trip camping our way through northern Victoria. Even though I was on my open licence, I hadn't needed to drive very often. Most times Alan had chauffeured me in our only car. The road trip was an opportunity for me to get some road hours up. *Think I need the return of my L plates*, I thought as I drove for almost the first time in two years. I had developed a tentative resistance to driving, almost a fear.

"If you drive then you can choose the radio station," Alan coaxed. He knew that I tired of listening to his choice of radio station. Alan liked to listen to horse racing and sport all the time. The sky was blue and the temperature warm for May. The road was straight with road works signs displayed along the shoulders. My body muscles loosened as I drove for some kilometres behind a sedentary slow caravan. "Pass it," Alan said, "It is going too slow."

I took a deep breath and drove towards the middle of the road to get a clear view of any oncoming traffic. It was a long straight clear stretch so I boldly pushed on the accelerator and took off onto the wrong side of the road, passed the car and caravan and reinstated my position on the left side of the two lane road way in front of the car that was towing the caravan. I felt empowered and successful. I relaxed into the driver's seat with two hands on the wheel. The window was open blowing warm air into the car, on this beautiful autumn morning. The car was packed with camping gear to almost the roof in the backseat. Trudy our newly acquired two year old German shorthaired pointer dog, was lying on top of our stuff, perusing the scenery from her vantage point. We were cruising away from the slow caravan and car behind us. My favourite Beatles song was blaring from the speakers when suddenly a hand crossed to the middle of the dash and changed the radio station to my worst nightmare, horse racing. "No, no it is my turn to listen to my choice of radio," I said rather aggressively. I was watching the road concentrating. I didn't need any distractions.

Without warning the car was skidding towards a white pole on the right side of the road. A voice in my head told to me to ease off the accelerator but under no circumstance reach for the brake. We were heading for a deep ditch beyond the white pole. Alan reached across and grabbed the steering wheel in an effort to turn the wheels towards the centre of the road. I was in a void, a place of silence until suddenly I felt my head being hit.

"Please stop," I begged though no-one came to help. The car stopped, leaning onto the driver's door. The engine was still revving. Alan ignored me, he was groaning. I loosened his seatbelt to make him more comfortable. I had to get help. A voice in my head told me to turn off the ignition and then I climbed through the empty space where the windscreen had once been. I had wrenched my feet from under the pedals leaving one shoe behind. I ran down the road to hail the car and caravan which had been following us. Tears cascaded down my face as I yelled, "Help me, please help me. Alan is stuck in the car, help me get him out." The car and caravan stopped. They were telling me to lie down on one of the caravan bunks.

"But I am fine. I just have a few grazes on my hand." I then realised that I was covered in what looked like my blood. It wasn't my blood it must be Alan's blood or Trudy's. I realised that Trudy was wedged between the roof of the car and my head, probably saving my life. She would have been so frightened. I looked towards the scene to see a semi—trailer driver working to get Alan out. With the help of some other car drivers who had stopped to help, Alan was taken from the car and attended to on the side of the road.

"There's a nurse on the scene. The ambulance is on its way." I overheard people around me saying. *Oh good he'll be fine once we get him out of the car,* I thought, *I don't need to worry about Alan now he's in professional hands. The nurse the ambulance the hospital doctors will all work to make him better because that is what they do.*

I suddenly realised that my dog Trudy was missing.

"What about my dog Trudy. She's gone." I cried.

"Don't worry about your dog worry about your husband," The woman from the caravan said sternly.

I overheard people saying that he was in good hands. It was all so confusing. Time passed very slowly until the ambulance arrived. The two Ambulance Officers engaged the help of a bystander to lift Alan and stabilise him in the back of the ambulance. The bystander seemed to be such a nice man. He asked me many questions about the accident.

We arrived at emergency in the nearest hospital where Alan was taken to surgery. I found that I had to negotiate with the doctor.

"I don't want an injection. Needles freak me out. I just need a cigarette. I'll be fine if I have a cigarette." My negotiation skills failed as I felt the injection pierce the skin on my thigh or somewhere around there.

"Smoking is not allowed in this hospital," he said assertively.

My brother Jake and my mother drove from Melbourne to Mildura to be with me. Alan's father and older brother drove to be with Alan. I didn't win the popularity polls with my in-laws needless to say. It was all too much to take in for everybody. *It was an accident and I was part of that accident. Why are they are being so cool towards me,* I thought. *This nightmare will end and I will wake up with all my dreams and future plans intact.*

The following day I made front-page headlines in the local paper. Thanks to the nice bystander my relationship with my in-laws decayed even further. The headline intimated that I was possibly speeding. Photos of the scene covered the front page that I held in my hand. That man who asked lots of questions was an evil journalist and a photographic journalist at that. He even sold a couple of photos to Alan's brother. I felt sick to the stomach and lit up a much needed cigarette. Nobody said a word, not even my mother who had tried to encourage me to give up the venomous smokes. I was very grateful to have Mum and Jake with me. I don't know what I would have done without them. They were there for me when Alan was airlifted to Melbourne without me. I felt even more transparent than ever. *Wasn't I Alan's wife of four years? Didn't that count for something? I know they said that there wasn't any room in the plane for me but what was I supposed to do?* I remembered the local paper's headlines. *The article made me look like I deliberately crashed the car. I wasn't speeding. Why did the journalist imply that I was? Didn't he realise that I was in the car too? Didn't he realise that it was my husband the other part of my life that was being flown away from me.* Alan was taken even further than I thought, he died two days later. When the doctor rang to tell me that Alan had passed on, I cried for Alan, and then I cried for me. Mixed feelings of sadness, guilt and hatred filled me. I felt bad when I thought about the newspaper article about our accident. The journalist had pointed his finger at me, painting a very black image of me I felt ripped off. *How could that man in the back of the ambulance trick me into believing that he was helping us?* Tears of rage poured down my cheeks. Then I thought of Alan, *poor poor Alan he was so young to have his life taken from him.* I hated God for stealing him from me which developed into feelings of resentment towards Alan for leaving me. Feelings poured through my being, making my head hurt, my eyes ache and my throat feel parched. *This is all too hard. I wish with every bone in my body that it was me who died and Alan who survived.* Alan was so much part of my life; he was all of my life. Losing Alan hurt too much.

I remembered talking to Alan about suicide when someone we knew attempted to take her own life. Her life as she knew it was running away from her. She needed the attention of the runner, to stop him and give her a sense of certainty that he would share the rest of their lives together. She was driven to do the worst, attempt to take her own life. Maybe she believed that it would be better for her to not be rather than be less significant in this man's life than she had been before. She wanted to be loved as she had before. Alan left this earth so suddenly and left me with a big hole in my life. The change was dramatic and my thoughts were chaotically running through my mind. I was doing a whole lot of overwhelm. It would have been so easy to go to sleep and not wake up, to not be here. It didn't seem fair that he had left me behind. I had to pull myself together and be strong. I didn't really know what being strong meant but I was determined to do it anyway. Think I was doing overwhelm and feeling unsafe. It was like the love of my life had abandoned me and then it was like he was taken away. Alan was my whole life and now he was gone.

I saw Alan's body laid out in his coffin. He looked so peaceful. There was a feeling of energy in the room as though Alan was above me filling the room with encouragement and peace. Alan's body was beautifully presented. His head obviously covered as a reminder of his injuries. Alan's pain was gone and mine dissipated momentarily. The space around me filled me with peace. My family were there for me. People expressed their sorrow for me but didn't really know what to say. Other people avoided me like I had the plague.

One of Alan's friends said to me quite bluntly, "I've met this special girl so I can't be seen being nice to you". I guess I had to make allowances for his youth which was evidently dominated by his testosterone marinated brain. I didn't fancy him I just wanted to be friends. At Alan's funeral one of his friends ignored me. I got the impression that he was angry with me. He turned away from me like he couldn't bear to look at me. I never saw this friend of Alan's again. Somewhere in the chaos of my mind it occurred to me that Alan's death was confronting and confusing for some of his friends. I too was facing up to bewilderment not understanding how such a tragedy could happen to me. I decided that I was going to be strong. I even decided that I would rely on my smokes for comfort and nobody would entice me into taking or using anything else. My smokes helped me think straight, or so I thought. I cried, I lost weight, and I smoked cigarettes. At times I felt like Alan was just away on holidays. I just wanted to write to Alan and tell him about those small issues of interest like, the house next door was rented that is why people came and went. They didn't bother to talk to us or form friendships because they weren't there long enough. But where would I send the letter. My tears fell to the ground.

Time passed so slowly, it was as if the pain stopped time. I couldn't for the life of me understand why God had taken Alan away from me. I wouldn't be turning to God for consolation. I told myself that I didn't want to feel restricted by rules with religion defining who I am to the world. I had escaped what I had experienced as the fundamentalist challenging religious world that I had been brought up in. I no longer wanted to be a sinner always grasping for forgiveness so I could be especially chosen to glow in righteousness. I would have to settle for just being a sinner. It was all too difficult and I didn't understand any of it. I just wanted to retrieve my life and continue those building blocks of life that Alan and I had planned for in the last year of his life. We were going to conquer the world with investments in real estate, travel through his work which would have enabled us to live in England and explore Europe. Then we planned a family to follow. We had plans to afford our children with a comfortable life as money and our love for each other would provide it all. I could picture these planning conversations so clearly. Memories of our adventures swept over me. I daydreamed about the good times that Alan and I had shared in more recent times where our relationship had changed from just sharing each other's company to planning for the future and enjoying each others company. My daydreams were so real I could feel Alan's excitement in anticipation just like I could feel the sun shining down on us with a breeze blowing as we walked through this new development that we were planning to invest in. These warm memories and experiences flooded through me. Other days I felt desolate.

"Why had Alan left me and not taken me with him. I felt so alone?" I cried out loud to empty spaces.

My work colleagues were very supportive. They gave me hope for a future as they encouraged me to begin again. One of them, Sandy organised a blind date. I agreed to consider going out on a blind date, even though in real time only a few months had passed. To me it felt like a lifetime since Alan and I were parted. My friends told me that at my age of 22 years old I needed to live and have fun. Sandy thought her daughter's future brother in law John was a gentleman and rather a good catch. In her mind he was waiting for just the right girl. In actual fact he was chasing women and a colour television. I was a woman and owned a colour television. The date was organised.

I froze when I heard the knock on the front door. My feet were stuck to the floor so my housemate opened the door for me. Melanie was thin and a little shorter than me with long dark hair falling freely to her mid back. Her blue eyes sparkled when she smiled showing a row of brilliant white teeth.

John looked at my house mate and burst into a huge smile.

"I'm here to take Anna out." She pointed towards me. The smile almost slipped from his face but he continued with his assignment.

John drove his monster green Fairlane car into the city. He found a free parking space a few streets from the theatre. My heart thumped as we trekked the city streets towards the movie theatre. The further we walked the more guilt consumed me. *What if my husband's family catch me out with another man?* I thought. Goosebumps filled my exposed skin, my heart thumped and my mouth dried. I just wanted to hide from the world. I thanked God that it was a dark moonless night and I probably wouldn't be recognised in the shadows anyway. John took me to see the Sound of Music on our first date. How could watching the Sound of Music be anything but angelic? John and I spent time together, sitting on the beanbags focusing on the colour television in front of us. My dog Trudy would sit behind us and growl.

"She doesn't like men, so don't worry about her." I assured John. I learned much later that it was only certain men who Trudy didn't like. I was too consumed with feelings of guilt about moving on. I didn't know the rules and I was frightened of being found out. There were some people who were not encouraging me to move on and those who were? I didn't know what I was supposed to do. I was afraid and torn between not knowing who I had to please and who would judge me. I had spent much of my life trying to please others and God in particular. My mind was filled with confusion around what to do there were times when I thought that Alan was the lucky one. I knew intuitively that I would have to make the best of what was left of the rest of my life because I made a belief that it would what Alan would have expected of me.

CHAPTER FIFTEEN

Within twelve months John and I became an item on paper, we were married. We had some fun experiences like camping and travelling overseas, but the foundation of our relationship was very unsteady. We married for the wrong reasons. He was motivated to meet his goal to be married by the age of 25. I was motivated to escape my fears around rejection and being found out as I was constantly worrying about what people would think or how they would judge me. We built a lot of emptiness in our relationship. My life with John was empty like I was surviving one day at a time. I filled my emptiness with colourful, loud drama. I built many more layers of emotions in my life, in an attempt to build a mask to hide behind so that I could please others who would like me for what they saw on that very top layer. It was just like I was applying many coats of paint to original building materials, to hide imperfections, to hide mistakes and to build a façade. I felt like I was part of John's façade, just like a handbag can compliment an outfit I believed it was my duty to be there to compliment him. Through mutual agreement this relationship was very short-lived. For some time I was unaware that I took from this relationship my layers of emotional baggage that I had built in my drama cycle, as a constant reminder of doing life hard.

A couple of months after my release from John, I met someone else who sparked a chord. He really did want to get to know me, warts and all. Tim would listen to what I had to say. We laughed together, we played together, we spent lots of time together and we both felt like we belonged together. There was lots of curiosity, honesty and learning in our relationship. Tim was curious to learn about me and I about him. I relaxed into this relationship where I felt wanted, loved and free to be me.

CHAPTER SIXTEEN

"I feel like throwing up. It's like this nausea feeling is part of me. I think *that I might be pregnant*," I told my work friend Joan, who was my friend and mentor. She had the experience of five pregnancies. Joan stopped typing and looked over the top of her reading glasses at me. I must have looked a little green and sickly. After some thought and observation Joan told me that whilst pregnant she would only hold food down for a matter of minutes after each meal.

"The doctor told me not to worry about throwing up. My system would absorb something in those few minutes, enough to nourish me anyway. I actually weighed less at the end of my pregnancies than I did at the beginning," said Joan.

I listened intently wondering how Joan coped for nine months five times. *How horrible*, I thought, *my nausea is intolerable*. Joan starred and broke into a smile and said, "You know Anna I think that you may be pregnant."

I spoke quickly, "This is amazing as I was told by an expert doctor that I wouldn't be able to conceive naturally."

My G.P. Doctor confirmed my pregnancy. Smiling broadly she said,

"Congratulations and you can have one glass of champagne to celebrate when you get home, but no alcohol after that at all during your pregnancy. Okay?"

"Yes. I can't tolerate too much anyway as I feel so sick. I can't even smoke, it disagrees with me even more," I said.

My Doctor was a mother, who with her Doctor husband ran the medical clinic. She smiled, "Feeling sick is good. There is no medication that I can prescribe to stop the nausea. You may find that eating small meals may help you feel better."

I didn't care about eating. I just wanted to tell Tim our wonderful news.

The butterflies were racing in my stomach. I knew that I needed to ring my mother. I dialled and listened anxiously to the ring tones. My heart was thumping. It felt like it was in my mouth.

"Hello," my mum's familiar voice said on the other end of the phone.

"Mum, I have news that you won't be happy with. It is okay if I don't hear from you while you think about it. I will tell you and then I will wait for you to ring me," I said very quickly. I took a deep breath and continued,

"I am pregnant."

I didn't hear from Mum for about two weeks. In her eyes, not only was I living in sin with Tim. I was also pregnant out of wedlock? It was more than her religious and culture beliefs permitted.

I knew my Mum would need time to deal with the information and two weeks later my Mum rang me.

Andrew arrived one day late. I was totally unprepared for his birth in spite of attending all the birthing educational classes available to me. I huffed and puffed and begged for help as the pain was all consuming. Then an epidural was inserted into my back giving me instant relief. I lay there while nature took its course not feeling very much at all.

Doctor Delicious was my recommended gynaecologist. He had been assessed by many women who knew women that I knew and they unanimously called him Dr Delicious. I could see why. He was tall, dark, handsome, drove a BMW car, and his smile would melt many a woman's heart. Dr Delicious arrived dressed in a long rubber apron which protected him from the tips of his toes to the top of his shoulders where they met his neck. He swished around the room looking very busy. He paused mid step and said, "Anna, you need to marry Tim. I think he's a really nice guy. Make sure you marry him."

I was in no position to disagree. *Doctor Delicious seems too smooth to be honourable*, I thought, *I wonder if his advice was thrown in for free or had he been speaking with my Mum?*

Dr Delicious spoke, "Quick nurse. We need to organise theatre and push the baby back up the birth canal to allow us to proceed with a caesarean section. The baby is too big for her disproportionate pelvic bones." Then he asked me, "Are you happy with going to surgery?"

"Well as long as you give me something so I don't feel the knife," I responded. His blue eyes twinkled and a smile ripped across his face when he said, "We'll give you a stronger drug in the epidural. I assure you that you won't feel a thing. Well you will probably experience a tugging sensation but that is all."

Andrew was born at 5am. I was proud of Andrew as he sat supported in the palm of the doctor's hand. His little face was scrunched like an old wise man's and then he pooped in the doctor's hand.

So he should, I thought to myself. *Poor baby has been through a lot*

Tim smiled through his fog of tiredness.

It was time to concentrate on me. I had an epidural, two drains, and a drip protruding from my body when I was wheeled from theatre.

"You'll need to have a kidney x-ray when they open the clinic next door to assure that I have repaired the bleeding damage which occurred during surgery," said Doctor Delicious. He left me in the nurse's care.

"I'll administer the Pethidine injection for when you have the kidney x-ray as it could prove painful," the nurse said.

I was grateful. I don't like pain. Finally it was time for the x-ray. I was wheeled in and left with one female radiographer.

"Can you slide onto the table for me?" she asked.

How I am going to do that, I thought. I couldn't move. My mind was willing but my body was like a dead lead weight.

"No," I said.

"Oh all right then," she snapped. "I'll have to find someone to help me" and she did. Fortunately everything was fine. I just had to be wheeled back to the ward to begin my recuperation. I waited for staff to bring Andrew to me. I was worried about how to hold him and how to look after him as I hadn't any experience with babies. Many hours passed when staff finally brought him to me.

"He is beautiful", I muttered. I learned very quickly how to feed, bath and take care of him. I took him home where I loved him and worried constantly about him. During my snapshots of sleep I would wake worrying that someone would steal him from me. Andrew was always there when I checked. With much ado I learned to breast feed. Breastfeeding didn't feel very natural and I missed not having my body just for me.

Where I lived in the suburbs of Melbourne the health department provided great services through its Health Centres for mothers with young babies. Life was a learning curve. Not only did I have to learn about mothering a totally dependent being. I also learned that Andrew's forefather, great great grandfather on Tim's side of the family, Sir George Cuscaden, established Baby Health Centre support for babies and mothers in Victroia. The Health Centre proved to be vital in its role in my life as a new mother. I followed the government's plan for visiting the Health Centre regularly with my new born. The Health Centre Sister told me that new mums needed to be super organised and have their babies asleep by six o'clock in the evening, in time for the father's return from work where he would become the centre of attention. Well that never happened in our household, Tim adored Andrew and enjoyed spending time with him.

Tim and I did decide to marry when Andrew was about five months old. We decided on a quiet home ceremony because we wanted to be married not so much get married. I did the right things and bought a new dress for the occasion and organised a session at the hairdressers. Andrew and I went to the hairdressers for me to have my hair styled and permed into the curly locks that were fashionable for the day. It was Monday and the first day of my planned week for wedding preparation activities. I planned to clean the house, prepare food in-between looking after Andrew whom I loved more and more as time passed.

"It's like he's always been part of my life," I told the hairdresser. Andrew was propped up in his pusher, watching people around him work.

He watched my hairdresser intently for a short while but that became a little boring so he cooed and giggled at anyone who would give him a spare second of attention.

"He's so cute," the hairdresser said.

"Yes he's beautiful but sometimes it's hard to know what to do to relieve his sore gums whilst he's teething." I told her.

"Well you just need to rub ouzo on his gums. That will help. My mother used ouzo on my gums when I was a baby." The hairdresser responded.

"Mmmm I like ouzo with coke," I said. *Ouzo on its own is a bit strong for me. It would knock Andrew for a six wouldn't it?* I thought

I changed Andrew's nappy soon after I got home. I was surprised to find a lump on the top of his thigh and thought that maybe his clothes were somehow rubbing him there. I decided to have it checked by the Health Centre Sister who quickly suggested I go to my family doctor. Thoughts of a hernia raced through my mind.

"Your doctor is on holidays. We will book you with the locum," The Receptionist said. I thought quickly, *I want to see my own Doctor. The locum doesn't know me or Andrew like my own Doctor does, but I will give it a go anyway. After all I am here now. The worst scenario is that I come back again when my Doctor returns.*

I agreed to let the locum doctor take a look at Andrew's leg just like the Health Centre Sister had instructed me.

It was our turn to see the Doctor. He smiled and said hello as we entered his room.

"Take a seat," He asked as he watched us. "How can I help you today?"

"Well my baby, Andrew has a lump on his thigh that I would like you to check. I don't know what it is. I have been to see my Health Centre Sister and she said that I should come and see you."

After careful examination he said, "You need to take Andrew to a paediatrician very quickly." He began to mumble or talk to himself like he was thinking out loud. "Andrew needs to see a specialist paediatrician."

He rang the specialist paediatrician whose rooms were close by.

The planning started in my head, I mumbled, "Tim will be home from work now. I'll drive past and collect him on the way through."

It seemed like only minutes had passed when Tim and I were greeted by the paediatrician who was waiting for us to arrive. He carefully checked Andrew, feeling and shining a torch through the area on his thigh where the lump appeared. He made small talk with Tim about the commonality of the old school tie. He excused himself whilst he made a phone call to discuss Andrew's lump with someone on the other end. Tim and I waited calmly discussing what we would have for tea. Our stomachs were grumbling telling us to feed them.

"You need to go to the Royal Children's hospital tonight. The Doctor will be expecting you." The Paediatrician stopped for breath and smiled kindly. He was dressed in a quality woollen suit with collar, tie and waistcoat. His hair was greying reflecting his maturity. I felt comforted and reassured in his presence. The Paediatrician continued, "Now I want you to go home and have some dinner then go into town to the Children's Hospital." We lived on the outskirts of Melbourne in the beautiful leafy suburb of Ferntree Gully. The Children's Hospital was on the other side of town about forty kilometres away, give or take a few kilometres.

Parenting was all so new to us. When we got to the hospital we were seen very quickly. It was seven o'clock in the evening at this stage of a very long day. The Specialist Surgeon was very patient and very caring as he carefully examined Andrew. I can't remember much more about the surgeon other than I trusted him implicitly. He sent us home with some prescribed anti-biotics. Fortunately the follow up visit on the Thursday before Tim and I were to be married would be in the specialist consulting rooms not far from where we lived. I breathed a sigh of relief when I realised that I wouldn't have to drive through the city to the hospital for the follow up consultation. Even though I had been driving for nearly ten years I feared driving in unknown territory with lots of traffic like there was in the City of Melbourne. The car crash that I had experienced in my previous decade lived with me fuelling my fear and undermining my confidence especially in relation to driving. The mere thought of driving in unknown territory triggered images to float around in my mind of the serious car accident I had nearly a decade before. Those images frightened me. They were constant reminders that within a split second I had lost control of the car with fatal consequences. It took a split second for my world as I had known it to no longer exist. It was much bigger than that feeling of losing your balance on a bike and falling to the ground. At least then I could get up shake myself and get back on my bike and take control to learn to balance. I was relieved to know that I would only have to drive Andrew and me in an area that was familiar to me. It was midnight when we finally lay our heads on our pillows to enter the world of sleep.

The following day I had to change my plans to add to the Tuesday list of things to do. My Thursday plans were reshuffled to fit in the Specialist visit. On Saturday Tim and I were going to be married at home. I hurried through my preparation of the house and accidentally locked sleeping Andrew in the house with me outside. I tried breaking in but to no avail. I had managed to break into other houses through windows or window screens, when I had locked the keys inside. This time the windows and door locks secured me on the outside.

"Andrew's inside. I can't leave him there by himself," I cried in panic.

I picked up a brick, threw it and broke the bathroom window, the smallest window in the house. The glass shattered and banged as it crashed to the ground. The power tools in the area stopped for a split second. It was as though the tradesmen working nearby listened and then started their power tools again. No one came to investigate or help me. Relieved that I wasn't going to be busted for breaking and entering, I climbed onto the window sill and through the window. Now I had another job to add to my list. I had to organise for the window to be replaced. It was suddenly Thursday and I just had the food and drinks to organise for Saturday's festivities.

Andrew and I visited the specialist for his appointment. The Specialist looked and felt the lump. The Specialist Surgeon wasted no time to tell me that Andrew's lump had grown bigger. Our plans were changed rather rapidly. He said, "I want you to be in the Children's Hospital in time for surgery tomorrow. You will need to get there by 9a.m."

I said," but I'm getting married on Saturday at 1o'clock. Perhaps I should postpone my wedding?"

He smiled and assertively said, "No. Getting married is too important we'll work around it. You should be out of hospital in time."

Early the next morning I sat in the driver's seat behind the steering wheel. I sensibly took deep breaths reassuring myself that I could do this drive. I reminded myself that I was drawing on that courage and love that I had inherited from my parents in my vehicle of life. They would have done the same for their children and did do the same by moving to unfamiliar territory. They had after all moved to the unknown across the world from Holland to Australia to give their children the best opportunity for the best life that they could give them. I wasn't thrilled about having to drive through the city of Melbourne during peak hour traffic. I could feel my chest tighten just by thinking about it. I decided that if I mapped and memorised my route before I left, the route would not be totally unfamiliar.

Sitting behind the steering wheel I was totally focused in the present moment. I was concentrating on the road ahead, manoeuvring the car to strategically change lanes as needed. I watched carefully for my planned turns, and followed my plan. When we were safely parked in the hospital's carpark I realised that I had talked my plan to Andy who gurgled away in the back seat. Andy was only four and a half months old but proved to be a wonderful travelling companion.

Andy was back in his hospital bed with his much loved teddy bear that his aunty Siri had given him. His little leg was bandaged which was the only sign of his adventure in the operating theatre. I slept in a chair beside his bed while nurses quietly observed him throughout the night. We were discharged on Saturday morning. In fact we arrived home one hour before Tim and my wedding proceedings were due to start and I hadn't organised the food. Though Tim had bought some food and the drinks, my sister in law Jill had kindly offered some of my nephew's sixteenth birthday party food and she made a wedding cake for us as a present. I felt so appreciative.

I was suddenly very nervous but the wedding went well and without a hitch. It was a small ceremony and family were asked to join us afterwards for an afternoon tea celebration. It is what we wanted. I was nervous enough with just the Celebrant, Tim and our witnesses. Any more people and I would have been a terrible nervous mess.

Monday morning happened very quickly and I was concerned about Andrew's wound. I needed to call the hospital to find out when I could bath him properly. The doctor's receptionist told me to treat it like any hernia operation and then virtually finished the conversation.

"She must have thought that we had previous experience with hernia operations," I said to Tim. "I guess we are older than many as first time parents. Most people start their families in their twenties not their thirties"

I had not long replaced the phone in its cradle when it rang again.

"Hello," I answered.

"This is the Specialist from the Hospital is Mrs Derham there please?" asked the voice on the other end of the phone.

"Yes speaking," I responded. The conversation suddenly became surreal.

"I'm sorry but it is a tumour." These words echoed through the phone line. I felt like I was gasping for air.

"You need to come into the hospital NOW."

CHAPTER SEVENTEEN

"The lump on Andrew's leg, it's a tumour," I said. I didn't wait for a reply. I quickly said goodbye to my sister in law Jill, replaced the phone in its cradle and left for the hospital.

Tim, Andrew and I found ourselves in the hospital's lift as we were to go directly to the surgical ward which Andrew and I had left only days before.

"I heard that you two were married on Saturday", said a nurse in the elevator.

"Yes, we were," I said

"Congratulations," She said

"Wow how did you know?" I asked.

"News travels fast here." She said, "I have to leave you on this floor. Good Luck with everything."

The specialist surgeon had organised for his secretary to escort us to the surgical ward. I felt reassured, well a little reassured that at least we weren't going to the cancer ward. Once Andrew was settled in his hospital bed Tim left to return to work. I settled into my chair beside Andrew's bed. I looked at my sleeping baby wondering why this was happening to such a little person and to me. It was happening to Tim to but it was all so overwhelming that I could only see the world from my map of my world. I decided I needed to talk to God. I told myself, that even though I had given up on God I would talk to him anyway. I sat beside Andrew's hospital bed and asked,

"God. Why are you doing this to me and my baby? What could Andrew have possibly done to you to deserve this? This whole deal is so unfair. We love Andrew and take good care of him and you want to take him away from me too. Haven't I experienced enough of life being taken away from me already?" I could feel the anger rise within me, I was really angry with God. My mouth was dry, but my hands were sweaty. My heart was pumping. On reflection it was like road rage but a God rage equivalent. I sat beside Andrew's bed watching him in disbelief. I loved him so much, "How could this be happening to him and to us?"

There were many tests and many doctors consulting. I lived in the hospital for Andrew's stay. I was almost relieved when Andrew was finally on his way to surgery. "There's surgery and then he will be on his way to getting better," I told myself, "We can do that."

The hospital staff were accommodating and I was given a bed in a room usually reserved for breastfeeding mothers of premature babies. It was a shared a room. I shared with a mother whose son was much older than Andrew with whom I participated in small talk. This friendly woman suddenly turned the conversation.

She asked, "Is Andrew's tumour a secondary tumour?"

I don't really know. I heard the term metastases but I didn't really understand what that meant and I have no clue what a secondary tumour is, I thought. She didn't wait for an answer.

"It's just that if it is a secondary, then it is curtains," she said as she lazed back on her bed locking her hands behind her neck for support on her lumpy pillow. I heard her voice wafting on and on, finally talking about her son's health. I just couldn't concentrate on the words.

I concentrated on the practical, focusing on my purse which I placed within reach of my bed. Tim had left me with a few dollars to buy something to eat for breakfast. It was like my purse was my comfort. I took my purse with me when the nurses called me to Andrew's bedside. I must have forgotten it on the last visit in the early hours of the morning. When I awoke in the morning my purse was gone. I reported the theft to the hospital security guards. We had our suspicions but couldn't prove anything. Just as well that I wasn't feeling very hungry. I told my room mate that my purse was missing. She looked at me and said again that if Andrew had secondary cancer, then he would certainly die.

"By the way did you take my soap from the shower? It's gone and it was a very expensive soap given to me by my boyfriend," She said accusingly.

"No I used my own soap." I said. "*Why would I use someone else's soap? Who knows what sort of germs could be on it. Oh who cares about soap at a time like this? Why was she being nasty towards me, she doesn't even know me?*" I thought.

Her words were unnerving, breaking my confidence that the doctors would heal Andrew. Panic set in making my heart thump and my head spin. I tried to tell myself that I should listen to the doctors not to her, but the doctors weren't giving much away at this point in time. I had thoughts of Andrew's imminent death dancing in my head. I tried to push these thoughts away but they lurked in the background.

We had just been transferred to the Cancer ward upstairs in six east, where I found myself following another mum into the kitchen to make a cup of tea.

"Are you participating in the full blown chemotherapy treatment?" the mum asked me.

"I don't know. I don't even know why I am here. My son has just been moved here from the surgical ward. I just don't . . ." My voice wavered.

"Oh um it's just that my daughter has already started her chemotherapy treatment, and I thought that your child had too."

"How's it going?" I asked.

"She's responding well and we're hoping that she will recover to live a normal life." And so the conversation continued.

Andrew had to have another operation to look at his kidney. The ultrasound tests showed an unusual growth near the kidney. Perhaps the muscle tumour, called something like rhabdomyosarcoma had spread.

It was time for Andrew to have his operation. He bravely went into surgery with his favourite teddy bear by his side.

The Surgeon visited Andrew's bedside. He was a kind man, insistent on informing us about our son.

"We removed the tumour which looked like it had grown beside the kidney. I removed the part of the kidney that was affected. On the spur of the moment I decided to take the whole kidney just to find that the part that I thought was good actually had a growth in it also." The surgeon was extremely honest and compassionate when speaking with us.

We didn't have to wait long before Andrew's Oncologist asked to meet with Tim and I in the briefing room. We learned that it was the same room that parents came to fear because this was often the room where the bad news was told.

The Oncologist said, "Andrew's cancer cells are not like other cells in his body. The cells are presenting as undifferentiated sarcoma because the mutated cells don't mimic any other cells in his body. Therefore the cancer cells are unidentifiable. We cannot recognise from where the cancer originates. However we did remove masses from the kidney. The oncology team believe that we should try treating Andrew's cancer with the chemotherapy treatment used for Wilms tumours." He continued to tell us that after Andrew's kidney was removed, the cancer name changed to a Rhabdoid Wilms tumour. Apparently in children Wilms tumours were the tumours more commonly found in the kidney?

"How long will Andrew need to be treated?" I asked

"We will constantly assess Andrew's progress but I would think that he will need at least two years of treatment. We believe that we can cure undifferentiated sarcoma but we don't know if we can cure your son. We believe that Andrew has a 10% chance of surviving this cancer," said the Oncologist.

Tim and I leaned into each other. Neither of us could stop the tears from falling. Two grownups sobbing proved to be too much for the doctor to deal with. He left the room asking the nurse to take care of us. The nurse spent time empathising and helping us to pull ourselves together to take the first steps to face the beginning of the rest of this journey.

It was discharge time. Andrew had been given his first dose of chemotherapy. We couldn't get out of the hospital quick enough. We so wanted to be back in the comfort of our own home. By the time we got to the car, in the hospital car park, Andrew had thrown up everywhere. It was incomprehensible and we were not prepared.

Every week on a Monday morning I would take Andrew into the hospital for his chemotherapy treatment. Andrew and I would line up in the corridor to see the oncology team who would refer us to the nurses next door for the next lot of chemotherapy. One day Andrew was so distressed that the veins in his head became very pronounced. There were problems finding the veins elsewhere because he was so small I guess. We were all upset that this had to happen but it meant that it was over quickly and the side effects were still the same. Andrew was so terribly sick, every day in fact. It was not unusual for me to change him four or five times per day. I would carry water and wool wash in the car. Nearly every trip I would clean the car's surfaces quickly to stop the smell inducing further vomiting.

One horrible day the lump in his leg reappeared. The Surgeon refused to put Andrew through any more surgery. Andrew was then treated with radio therapy treatment at Peter MacCallum Cancer Centre to reduce the size of the lump. At least he didn't have to have chemotherapy during this time. Andrew's energy levels dropped quite substantially from the added stress placed on his little body. The doctors ordered a blood transfusion, which brought the colour back into his face.

"He just looks better but he isn't," said The Oncologist. He clearly didn't want us to get our hopes up.

Andrew appeared to be a little stronger after the blood transfusion. He needed some strength to deal with the radiotherapy sessions. These treatments were about reducing the lump it was not about curing his cancer. I took Andrew's Journey day by day. My main concern was to help him feel as comfortable as I possibly could. I didn't allow myself to think past the present moment. I was getting the message that some people thought that I was in denial. A young radiographer looked me in the eye and asked, "How many bedrooms did you say you have in your house?"

"Four," I replied

"Well you should work on filling them," She said with saddened eyes filled with heartfelt compassion.

I heard but didn't really listen. I was about giving Andrew the best chance at life that I could. The stress took its toll. My back started to hurt so much that I couldn't stand straight. A visit with the chiropractor on a Saturday morning would fix it. My chiropractor had just stopped working Saturday mornings. He suggested that I visit his brother Peter who was also a chiropractor.

"I have a baby son and he has cancer." Peter stopped. He thought about what I said looked at me directly and asked, "You have cancer?"

"No my baby, my baby Andrew has cancer," I sobbed. After a short silence he took charge and told me of a seminar with Dr Anne Wigmore at Melbourne University the following day. He thought that she may be able to help us.

The next morning Tim, Andrew and I drove forty or so kilometres into the middle of Melbourne to attend the Dr Anne Wigmore seminar at Melbourne University. To my surprise, my very new chiropractor Peter was there as well. Peter had a big Saturday night, the night before. He and his family were celebrating their new home whilst farewelling their current neighbours. Peter said," I didn't know whether you would come. I needed to gather information for you."

I thought. *"Wow he doesn't really know us, but he cares enough to research options for our son"* I was taken aback by his kindness and concern.

We learned about wheat grass and how to grow it, how to make smoothies with fruit and vegetables and what to eat to help battle cancer.

"You know Peter this will be good for you after a night partying," I said tongue in cheek.

"You know you are right," he said, "That red wine certainly leaves its side effects. After some tasting here today I should feel really well." Peter smiled, and continued, "There's a young man who wants to come and talk to you about options. He knows a doctor (a Professor now) who he believes will be able to help you." Our Cancer Journey was taking a turn of hope.

The Professor took hair analysis samples from me and from the little amount of hair left on Andrew's head, to find the deficiencies in both Andrew and my diets. I was breast feeding him and that's all he could eat. I needed to follow a new eating and supplement regime to afford Andrew the best chance to provide him with a whole food through my breast milk. Vitamin C, Selenium and antioxidants were given as supplements and I was to eat organically grown food, grow and juice wheat grass.

Through the synchronicity of talking to the young man at the Anne Wigmore seminar we had in fact unleashed international help for our son, through our new medical contacts we received a special supplement from a clinic in Switzerland and advice from an oncologist in Germany who asked for a copy of Andrew's medical history to be sent to him in Germany.

Andrew's Oncologist appeared to me to be quite taken aback when I requested a copy of Andrew's history. In my mind Andrew's Oncologist spoke to me in a condescending tone and I remember him saying that if I were looking at alternative therapies then I was just wasting my money. When I told him that it was for an Oncologist and Physicist in Germany, Andrew's Oncologist had the information in my letter box by the next day and a copy was sent to Germany as well. That was the last that I saw of what I determined to be Andy's Oncologist's condescending manner.

Our next port of call was a visit to Ian Gawler's healing sessions.

"We have a new session starting soon. Why don't you both come along for the first session?" said Ian. My mind was scrambled from tiredness and I didn't realise that he meant Tim and I, not Andrew and I. Nevertheless Andrew loved being there amongst all those people who were learning about the power of creative visualisation and meditation and how to use it to heal. He gurgled and smiled at people and reached out for anyone who would give him attention. Without warning Andrew screamed in pain as he was being burned by his own digestive system. It was like his medicine or illness was changing his molecules into toxic burning acid. Andrew screamed. All I could do was clean him up, change his nappy and try to soothe him.

The chemotherapy treatment recommenced at the conclusion of radiotherapy treatment. There would be no reprieve as a pause in chemo treatment would render it ineffectual. It was not long before Andrew's Oncologist met with Tim and me for another meeting. We followed Andrew's Oncologist down the hallway to the bad news room. Andrew's Oncologist said,

"Chemotherapy treatment will not cure Andrew but we don't have anything more to offer him." Andrew's Oncologist paused and watched the tears pour down our faces. He paused for a moment and then continued,

"We are at the point where you need to decide whether to continue chemotherapy treatment for Andrew. It may increase his time that he has left or it may not. We cannot make any promises or give you any guarantees. At this stage some families decide to continue the chemotherapy and other families decide not to."

I asked, "Can we give Andrew a break from the treatment while we think about it?"

Andrew's Oncologist said, "Andrew can miss one week's treatment but any more time and chemotherapy will not work for him again. That's the nature of his chemotherapy. That is all we have to offer." Tim and I decided to cease Andrew's chemotherapy treatment in the hope that he would have some time with us where he wasn't throwing up, where he wasn't burning up. We decided to cease chemotherapy treatment.

"What do you mean that you will make a decision about whether Andrew continues his chemotherapy? Who do you think you are making decisions like that?" My long time Doctor's voice was rising in decibels with each word spoken. The same Doctor who had told me to go home and celebrate with one glass of champagne when she confirmed my pregnancy.

Tim carried Andy and we walked from the doctor's surgery in a daze.

"I thought that she would be supportive, not rip strips off us. She's been my doctor for years. She has been with me through my life's ups and downs. It's like she is abandoning me when I need her the most." I said to Tim.

I think I was in shock. I was certainly suffering from disbelief, building yet another layer of experience to deal with. I never went back to her again.

We continued with the strict regime of eating healthily and taking the supplements. Now we had visits to the Professor as well as the hospital, though the hospital visits were further apart. The hospital visits were now just for examinations just to keep an eye on Andrew's progress.

Andrew stopped smiling and lost some of the little strength he had. He was never able to sit up by himself. Not long before Andrew's first birthday I noticed that he was stiffer than usual. I called the Professor but he wasn't available, consequently a Locum came to the house. The Locum sat in our lounge room. He assertively told us to, "ring the hospital and let them know that you are coming in now. I will not leave here until I know that you are in that car on your way to the Children's Hospital."

Our dinner plates with their half eaten meals were left just sitting on the dining room table until our return sometime in the future.

When we arrived at the Royal Children's hospital in Melbourne a doctor and a neurologist were waiting for us. Surgery was scheduled for the next day to put a shunt into Andrew's head to drain excess fluid. In preparation they gave Andrew a scan only to find that he had a huge brain tumour and that meant that the end was very near. Sadness pressed heavily on me and on Tim. A voice inside me, an irritant, reminded me that Andrew wasn't christened. When I felt let down by God I made a vow that no child of mine would be christened. Somewhere deep inside I needed to know that I had done whatever I could for Andrew. The only thing left was his spirituality. He was too young to make his own decisions. I had a responsibility to do it for him. Tim organised for his Vicar to come to the hospital to perform a christening. He would be christened Church of England. Afterwards I felt a weight lift from my shoulders. So much for hating and blaming God for this dreadful experience that Andrew had to endure. God would soon take Andrew from me and care for him. My belief in God had changed or had I just found God again as a God who didn't scare me anymore. I was beginning to change my perception and belief around God to that of a loving God who would keep Andrew safe when he passed on. I trusted that God would do that for Andrew and that is why I wanted to have him christened. I knew then that I believed in God. It was like God had transformed his energy into a loving God who would care for Andrew. A Catholic friend of the family told me that babies who die become angels. In my mind Andrew would always be an angel.

Back on earth Andrew was given steroids and valium along with other medication to reduce swelling and help with pain. Andrew lay in my arms, his breathing laboured and his head was growing bigger as we watched. The tumor was consistent in doubling its size. I felt a need to hold his head and support his body. His little body became disproportionate. His head lay heavily against my arm. When I shifted I noticed that the area around his ear was turning blue. I gave him to Tim to share the nursing. Andrew's breathing laboured. There was a sombre mood in the room that was interrupted with a sharing of humour. Andrew opened his eyes and I swear I saw him smile for the gift of humour and then he took his last breath. I felt relieved that Andrew was free but the hole he left in my heart hurt and came with an intensity I could never have imagined. This pain eased with every hour that passed. As one forgets the pain of giving birth so it felt that I was forgetting the intensity of pain with my little man's death. I was a little distracted with the physical pain and feeling sick from medication to dry up my milk. I couldn't go back I could only go forward. *I can do this I have recovered from loss before I know I am tough,* I thought.

Family and friends were there to support me. I hadn't even thought how Andrew's passing would have affected those around me. I have no idea why but I thought it was my burden to bear for me alone. Perhaps I blamed myself somewhere deep inside me. I had alienated myself from everyone without even realising it. After all it was Tim and my loss. I didn't think that others were hurting too. I failed to see that the death of someone so young would touch so many people. The tragedy of Andrew's death in my mind was incomprehensible and unjust.

I busied myself carefully packing Andrew's clothing and belongings. I could smell him and sense him in his room. I loved him so much that when I stopped being busy I became present to my pain of loss which was still intense and excruciating but a little less than it had been as each hour passed. I had to get busy again. I had to deal with Andrew's stuff quickly before the hurt numbed me. I finished his photo album, the only tangible memory that I had of Andrew's existence.

Time was racing we would soon say our final goodbyes. The pain was still intense but easing with time.

I'm not wearing black, I thought to myself. The tears were leaking down my face, *I know it's respectful and traditional to wear black but I'm not going to. I don't care what people say or think. No one is going to force me to wear black.* Looking in the mirror I approved of my reflected image. I was wearing white, black was so sombre. The skin on my ankles, arms and face almost blended. It was like my blood had drained from my body and I was functioning on remote control. I couldn't feel. I could just see. The big black car collected Tim and me from home. I was in a time warp as it seemed only seconds before we were in the church which was more like a cathedral in the inner suburbs of Melbourne. Andrew's small white casket took centre place at the front of this awesomely big church. Tears poured down my face, I couldn't stop crying. The celebration of his short lived life was about to continue at the cemetery. I was walking past the flowers lining the church steps when I saw the humorous sight of my best childhood friend kissing my Dad. He was ashen as he clearly didn't recognise this young woman with multi coloured hair dressed in unfamiliar super trendy clothing. I could see that the tears stopped falling from his eyes as he lapped up the compassion from this unknown young woman. He asked much later, "Who was she?"

"Liz" I said. Dad's face had burst with emotion and a small smile. Liz had a spot in my Dad's heart.

Tim and I sat silently in the back of the car looking out through the darkened windows. Daily life continued on the outside, totally oblivious to our loss. We stepped out of the car onto the cemetery ground. Tim and I clutched each other closely; we froze, our legs threatening to give way beneath us. Tim's younger brother gently put his strong supporting arms around us and led us to the graveside where we watched the tiny casket with Andrew's little body being lowered gently to its resting place. We placed red roses on top of the coffin and said our last goodbyes. I knew then that Andrew would live on in our hearts forever.

CHAPTER EIGHTEEN

Ten months later the second of our four sons was born. I heeded Andrew's Paediatrician's advice, "Stay away from doctors unless you need to see one. The chances of cancer happening again are greater but still very slim. Well done with your addition to your family and enjoy."

I joined the new mothers' group at the local health centre where we met with our babies each week for the first six months of our babies' lives. We had moved to Ferntree Gully at the foot of the Dandenong's where we lived in a close supportive community which provided support for mothers of young children from babyhood to school age kids. Playgroups happened at the health centre preparing the kids for kindergarten in the building next door. Our playgroup sessions finished during kindy playtime. We could often hear the kids play talk as we walked to our cars. The kindergarten's play gym lined the back fence of the car park.

"Don't you speak to me like that you naughty boy." said a young four year old girl with finger wagging to another child climbing the ladder of the cubby.

"If I have to speak to you again I will put you in your room." She continued with finger still wagging.

"I wonder who she is modelling," I said to one of the playgroup mums as we walked towards the car. We smiled, looked at each other and said almost in unison, "I wonder if we sound like that."

How often do we look at ourselves in a true light and see what we are really doing. I want to be a new age mother guiding my children to have the freedom of choice in their lives, not be constrained by strict rules like I was. But you know what I could see myself in the kindy kids scenario. I am not sure about the finger wagging though, I thought walking to my car with my second born.

My life would entwine with these mothers from the new mothers group. I was part of their community and my family and I belonged to this community. Our community was close and small, fringing the beautiful Dandenong's in Victoria, where the air was fresh, the gum trees were tall and the blackberries were a pest.

CHAPTER NINETEEN

Life was happening to me. I had two young children, two boys and a husband so that could be three boys to look after. I was working part time, managing a house and a fairly full social calendar when my back started to hurt again. On one of my more regular visits to my Chiropractor, Peter, he suggested that I look outside the box and try something different to value add to his services.

I was about to embark on the most significant turning point of my life.

"There is a Silva seminar happening in the city in the Exhibition Building in town which I believe will help you. There are a couple of people I'm recommending the Silva program to because I think that it will help. I've done the course and believe that learning relaxation techniques will really help with your back pain management. In fact creative visualisation has been a tool used for attracting success in the workplace, healing of the mind and body, and contemplation of problems to raise awareness of choices that are available to everyone in life. I believe it will help you too." Peter handed me the invitation to the information session. This information had a familiarity, taking me back to Ian Gawler's session where he was teaching meditation techniques for many cancer sufferers. Ian had moved his sessions from the house in the suburbs into much larger premises in the rural outer suburbs of Melbourne to cater for the demand. *In my mind increased demand for meditation supports its credibility. There must be something in it, I* thought.

Obedience prevailed and the money to pay for the seminar came to me in part of a lump sum payout from my long service leave payout when I resigned from my job. I had decided that it was time to dedicate to being a fulltime mother. Our family had grown two healthy boys and later our bonus third bouncing bundle would arrive.

My friend Sue who worked in the library with me had an insatiable interest in psychology and how the mind works. Sue was very keen to accompany me to the information night and then later she and I participated in the Silva Mind Control program together. We completed the first Silva Mind Control program with a qualified psychologist facilitator. I learned to access more of my brain through creative visualisation. Through the process I was discovering a greater understanding of myself and those around me. It would be my first major step towards shifting to taking responsibility for my life instead of just letting life happen to me. Practicing my learned Silva meditation and creative visualisation techniques helped to dissipate my back pain. It was a win win win situation. I felt happier, my back wasn't hurting and my family got to experience a happier me.

There were times when I meditated that I felt a peacefulness envelope me. I think that I had discovered a little of what my mum would have liked to discover. I imagine that my Mum may have experienced the same peaceful feeling when she prayed. Mum did talk dreamily about discovering true peace, joy and love when God selected you to be one of his chosen few. I was discovering through practicing those Silva techniques that resonated with me that peace was already within me.

I subsequently discovered that peace, joy and love wasn't something earned but is the stillness that is inside me. I chose to generalise that we all have this awareness within us but we don't all choose to acknowledge it. I didn't share this supposition with my Mum. I assumed that I would only upset her if I shared my new findings with her, especially the bit where the idea of God energy being within us all was mooted.

I used my newfound meditation skills each day where I would relax and then visualise a healthy back, which helped me manage my pain. My new found meditation skills complimented my regular chiropractic maintenance checks. These new skills had elements of familiarity. I remembered an acquaintance who was an insurance salesman say that he had a picture of a BMW convertible posted on his office wall to motivate him towards achieving his dream in his career. He said that it was his dream to own a yellow BMW and that the picture would motivate him to take the action to get the results that he needed to buy his dream car. He said that it helped him to daydream to see a clear picture of the car, to smell its interior's newness, to imagine that he could hear its engine purring sweetly as he flattened his foot on the accelerator. He said that in his daydreams he would feel what it was like to caress the new upholstery and sit comfortably in the driver's seat. Every time that he saw the picture of his BMW on his wall he would imagine himself driving it as if it were his. He said that if he did this regularly he would take the steps to reach his goal, to be the proud owner of a BMW exactly like the picture on the wall.

I successfully used these brain exercising strategies to help me manage my study towards a library degree between working part time whilst being a wife and mothering three young children. I would begin by relaxing my body, and then I would relax my mind sitting in stillness momentarily. With a clear mind I would imagine myself effectively reaching the desired outcomes for the tasks that needed to be completed for that study period. I passed every subject some better than others.

I did however think that I had the cleanest toilets in the universe. When the adventure of my studies overwhelmed me I would need an escape to do something I knew how to do and that was cleaning our toilets.

"You know when study gets to boring or overwhelming one needs a distraction and mine is cleaning the toilets," I told my friend Sue, who frowned and just shook her head in disbelief.

I made a belief that my meditation or stillness helped to balance my study life between overwhelm and self empowerment.

My self awareness journey had begun but it seemed very slowly. Talking about my new found knowledge was laughed at by some and discredited by others. I knew that I could creatively visualise and that's when good things started happening for me. I remembered the Silva facilitator saying,

"The Silva program is about living in the present, processing for future abundance using creative visualisation and positive thinking." I sometimes found the stillness, but I was still vulnerable to stressful situations that I placed myself in. I searched for abundance and received good things sparingly.

Sometime later my friend Sue attended repeat sessions of the Silva program where she was told that it was essential to face your demons, but I didn't take it on-board at that time.

I later found The Secret which talks about night time car travel where you only see a couple of hundred metres ahead illuminated by the car's headlights. Even though you cannot see your destination you know that it lies ahead. You trust in the knowledge that you are travelling towards your destination and that keeps you driving even though you only have two hundred metres ahead of you illuminated. I made it mean that is where I was on my life's journey, learning to trust that I would get there. I was going forward not backwards where I would have to deal with my past.

Tim had been away from work for three months as illness after illness dug its claws into his system. Clearly he was stressed and life wasn't coming together for him in the beautiful foothills of the Dandenongs. The previous year we had entertained the idea of moving to Queensland. This time we needed to change something to ease our financial state of affairs, to afford our family a better quality of life. We spent much of our leisure time reading Qld newspapers and looking at Queensland house prices. Within three months we had sold our house, purchased another house just north of Brisbane but south of the Sunshine Coast. Tim had bought a business and we were on our way to a new beginning.

CHAPTER TWENTY

"Have a look at this job Anna. It's a casual library assistant position close to home," Tim said.

It sounds like a good opportunity to mix with other working people in an area that I know. It is only a casual library assistant position how binding can that be. I could fit in a couple of hours of work. I really like staying home with my kids but we could do with the money, I thought.

I had met quite a few people through the local church's play group. I even attended craft and self-development workshops run by the church. The most significant one that I attended was a personality profile workshop.

"You are a Sanguine personality. You like to have fun and enjoy people's company and dealing with other people," said the convener.

I thought about that for a moment then said, "Yes I agree. I'm amused that I'm a Leo though which means I'm a leader. I couldn't lead if my life depended on it."

The Convener quickly said," You may surprise yourself. If you were to find yourself in that situation you would probably do very well."

I was flabbergasted. The next day I attended the interview for the job. Before I went in I remembered the advice I had received the day before. *I could be a leader. I wonder if they would put me in charge of children's services in the Branch*, I thought dreamily. My mind cleared as nervousness took centre stage. I was so very nervous and told the panel so.

At least this time I'm only shaking, I haven't lost my voice through fear like I have done in past interviews, I thought to myself.

The interview was drawing to a close when I was asked,

"If you were to be the successful applicant would you be prepared to study and gain a degree in Library studies?"

"Yes I have been looking at upgrading my library technician qualification to a degree qualification through Charles Sturt University." I responded.

"Would you be prepared to be in charge of the Branch Library?" Reactively I was going to say no but I remembered the previous day's workshop and said yes.

After the interview I just wanted to get as far away as I could from the interview space. I was feeling very self conscious like I had made a fool of myself. I wasn't feeling terribly confident.

Well I got the job and studied part time for four years to get the coveted Library degree juggling work, study and home. I used my Silva meditation and positive thinking skills learned to get me through it. My new job was challenging. During my four years away from libraries, computers and technology had made major inroads affecting all aspects of library work. The expectation from younger staff was that I should know every aspect of library work even though I had been away from all the changes for such a long time, well a lot changes in four years. *Wow pressure*, I thought, *but I can do this*. I loved the idea of learning and knowing through osmosis but for me osmosis has never been. The challenges increased. I was a Branch Librarian of a new branch library facing the usual management challenges with humps to climb over. Stress intensified as quickly as change happened both on the work front and at home.

The phone call that most of us have to face sometime in our lives happened. It was my brother Jake. His voice wavered, "Anna, it has happened. We found Mum in her bed. Mum passed away during the night. We were visiting to have coffee with her. The ambulance was called. They did everything they could." I felt for Jake having to deal with it all. It seemed like no time had passed from the phone call till I flew to Melbourne for Mum's funeral. I was pleased to see Jake who met me at Tullamarine airport where we took time out to have a coffee. "Hey Anna did you have a good flight," Jake asked with interest.

I smiled and said, "Yes it was a good smooth flight. Thankfully I didn't get sick."

"Would you like to visit Dad first?" Jake asked. I missed my Dad. He was cared for in a dementia nursing home in the south east of Melbourne. I felt sorry for him as he seemed to me to be stuck in the atrocities of the Second World War. On previous visits I would watch helplessly as the bones in his face would contort stretching his thinning skin to opaque. His false teeth wobbled with every mouth movement as he babbled mixing Dutch with English. It wasn't unusual for Dad's eyes to fill with tears, whilst he spoke frantically, randomly throwing in the word Nazi.

We met Dad in the recreation room at the nursing home. He was sitting in his chair gazing at the garden through the big bay window. An English lady who volunteered her time to help in the nursing home stopped to talk to me.

"I don't understand a word your father says but I sense his anxiety." She said.

"Oh he speaks Dutch. But he does mix his English and Dutch beginning his speak midway through his thoughts," I said.

She thought for a moment before responding, "Oh so he's Dutch. That explains his agitation. The other day he became agitated when the nursing staff sat him in front of the window to watch the demolition of the old buildings. Your Dad had tears rolling down his cheeks. I quickly turned his wheelchair away from the window. He seemed to settle then. I guessed it must have reminded him of the bombings during the Second World War."

The English lady continued, "I remember the bombings in London," she said catching her breath before continuing, "My husband received good care in this nursing home. I was so appreciative of the way he was looked after that I continued to offer my services on a voluntary basis. I recognised your Dad's fear where others were just confused."

Later that day during the sombreness of mum's funeral I listened to her Minister telling us about hellfire and damnation. A friend sensing the macabre of the fundamentalist service turned to me and whispered,

"I can't help thinking of your mum's image with her legs sticking out the top of her small freezer that time she fell in head first and then slipped to the bottom. I'm sorry I should be serious" It wasn't funny that Mum broke her arm but we could see the humour of the situation after the doctors repaired her. We laughed when told about it after it happened and enjoyed a giggle breaking the sombre atmosphere of Mum's funeral. The service was what she requested but more than some of us could take. The Minister hardly mentioned Mum. He was on a mission to scare the living shit out of us, talking about our sins and where we would end up if we didn't repent. At times like that I wished we were born Catholic, at least then you only had to go to confession once a week and all was forgiven. I had too much to repent for.

I had buried my child and my husband. I felt a peace around them in their passing. Maybe I could rely on them to share that peace with me. My Mum often said that she worried about me. I remembered her telling me on my fortieth birthday how I reached an age where gravity would force everything downwards from hereon in and more importantly she still worried about me. I was out of control. Well yes I was out of control I no longer went to her church. She feared for my eternal life. Mum would no longer have these worries about me.

Earlier that day Dad had been dressed in his morning suit the same suit that he wore when he married mum nearly sixty years before. Dad didn't make it to Mum's funeral service though. He collapsed just before getting into the car at the nursing home.

The next day I visited Dad and fed him his last meal whilst he wept.

"She's gone, she's gone," he cried, in between each mouth full of food. Through the confusion of his dementia, he let me know that Mum was gone from his life. He cried muttering words like they have taken her.

"They have taken her away," he said repeatedly crying even harder. My sister in law Jill tried to console him, "Dad you still have us," she said.

Through the tears pouring down his cheeks he said very clearly, "But you've all gone over the creek."

Well he was right. Sjanie lived in the U.S., Matt had been teaching in Hong Kong and I lived in Queensland, many hours drive from Melbourne.

Jake would however spend as much time as he could with Dad, often settling him at night. On his way home from work Jake would make a detour to spend time pushing Dad in his wheel chair so that he could sit beside the busy road in front of the nursing home to watch the cars go by. It seemed to me that this image of cars on the road before him would distract the images revolving through his head of the Second World War which it seemed to me had become his reality. I reckon he needed distraction to sleep peacefully.

Even though Dad lived in a different reality he knew that Mum had passed away. His distress and his comment about feeling abandoned indicated to me that he didn't want to be abandoned. Maybe he even wanted to be with mum. One week later we buried Dad. He had fallen out of bed, broken his hip, and then developed pneumonia. Within one week my Mum and Dad were both taken from me. My siblings and I were orphaned.

Life continued. I returned to work busying myself, doing the same things that I always did. I leapt back into study dictated by necessity of meeting timelines not through choice. My lifestyle allowed just bits and pieces of time for me to feel sad, change was rapid and life was busy. We had sold our beautiful Queenslander and now lived in our newly built brick veneer on a glorious bush block surrounded by designated koala territory. Kangaroos would sit across the road and stare through our window. They seemed close enough for us to touch though they weren't. The kangaroos were smart enough to keep their distance. I wondered if they enjoyed staring at us as much as Tim and I liked staring at them. Tim and I share a love for wildlife. One Saturday morning when I returned home from work I was greeted with Tim excitedly pointing at a tree in our backyard, "Look at the tree," Tim yelled excitedly. He pointed to an aged gum tree trunk. I scanned the tree, looking at bark shedding and leaves swaying in the breeze. The trunk had a continuous stain like someone had dripped the honey jar down one side. Tim's face almost burst with a smile.

"It's koala pee. We have koalas in the backyard," He said excitedly.

"I love koalas, have you seen any," I asked just as excited.

"Yes just up there in the fork. Follow the big trunk until it forks then the first branch and you can see him behind the leaves.

I remembered when I was fifteen how I cried for endangered koalas when sitting in a car with my sister Sjanie and my brother in-law Marvin. We were speeding away from a huge Victorian bushfire burning through the Grampians. "The koalas won't know where to go and how to get away from the fire. I just want them to follow us." I sobbed.

Koalas in our backyard were a drawcard for some German friends to come and visit. The koalas must have known because they hid where we couldn't find them. We had the pee stained trees to show our German friends though.

This place, our new home, was magical. We had lots of gum trees and wildlife outside our backdoor. Inside was proving to be rather mystical too.

"I'm playing with Andrew," retorted Sam.

"Does he visit often?" I asked

"Yes every day," said Sam

"He must really like you," I said. "Can you see all of him?"

With furrowed brow he glared at me in disbelief," Of course I can."

Sam was our youngest and was yet to reach four years of age. Andrew's visits would be our secret.

The months were flying by and it was another new year when we were looking forward to my friend's Sue's yearly visit.

Early the next morning we were enjoying breakfast outside on the wide verandah when Sue became very serious and said, "I don't know whether I should tell you this but I went to a clairvoyant."

How perceptive, I thought. Somewhere deep, very deep inside I could hear my mother objecting to that practice which wasn't Christian. My recall was that my Mum used clairvoyant and sinful in the same sentence which for me equalled fear of retribution. I still had the fear somewhere inside me of good versus evil. It was like my thoughts of warning were protecting me from my fear of hellfire and damnation. *I don't need to feel that fear anymore, I thought to myself.* My curiosity had got the better of me. I smiled in agreement.

Sue continued, "The clairvoyant told me that I had a close friend whose son died. He likes his brothers and likes to play with them." I was gob smacked, the hairs on my arms and legs stood on end. I felt like the fear of psychics and the power beyond us had left my life, well almost. I remembered that Sam in his innocence had often talked about Andrew's visits and how they played games in the hallway. With age, Sam's perception of his world changed to the point that the white presence would later frighten him and then disappeared altogether.

Knowledge of Andrew's visits shook my inherent black and white perception and beliefs of life. *Respect electricity. Don't let little fingers poke at live power points,* echoed in my mind. "I know I can't see electricity but I have a healthy respect for it. Of course we know it can kill because we believe it will and dead electrocuted people have been seen." I said to the walls of my bathroom.

"Andrew's visits were real. Just like electricity we just can't see it." I beamed imagining that the beam illuminated my reflection in the mirror on the bathroom wall.

"You know what, it is just like air we can't see it but take it away from us and we would be left gasping and then shrivelled." I did feel less restricted and allowed myself to be curious and open-minded about that which wasn't tangible.

Some years later I attended a team building weekend workshop organised through work. We participated in team building activities as a group and then we were divided into smaller groups. The leader was a psychologist and through these sessions she determined that she needed to ask me, "Have you dealt with your son's death?"

"I don't know. What does it mean to deal with it? How will I know that I have dealt with it?" I asked her. I had heard the dealt with term before but I had no clue what it really meant.

"Make an appointment to come and see me." She said. She seemed to care and I needed someone to care. At that time in my perception of my world it seemed like everyone was extracting from me. I was a mother at home and a team leader at work, so of course people demanded stuff from me.

I attended a couple of sessions with the psychologist where I talked and learnt about building walls between me and others to protect me from taking on other people's energy. I could relax and visualise myself building a wall. I wasn't a very good bricklayer as I still managed to take other people's energy on board. I hadn't learnt what 'to deal with it' meant.

I would sit comfortably, relax, close my eyes, and do a 3 to 1 count whilst concentrating on my breathing. Most mornings I would visualise me working in my job doing the activities for the day ahead. Some mornings my mind would wander from my organisational visualisation. I would imagine that I was on an adventure, where I left boredom behind me. I would dream that I had a sense of being valued, of doing important work fulfilling other peoples' needs. I would see people around me smiling and laughing with me, even thanking me. There was lots of warm inviting colours flashing by, I could see people in colourful clothing, creative people who were laughing with me, thanking me for providing them with a fun experience. I could see artists hanging their art high on the white walls around us. My environment was filled with beautiful colours, where I was enjoying myself with others laughing and having fun. I felt like I was in a place where I belonged and where I was appreciated. Sometimes my mind would wander even further into my imagination where I could hear the sound of waves gently breaking on the sand. I sensed that I could taste the salt air and smell the seaweed, pungent smelling seaweed. I was the only one on the beach with just my dogs. They were chasing each other in and out of the water. I left these beautiful dreams feeling calm and energised for the day ahead. I invariably felt better about facing my day at work.

Late one winter's evening the phone rang. "Hello." I answered.

"Hi Anna. It's Liz here." Liz and I had been friends since we were eleven years old. We lived across the road from each other in Melbourne. We had retained a friendship sailing in and out of each others lives for the last forty or so years. Liz continued, "There is a library position being advertised in the Whitsunday Times. I remember you telling me when you were here on holidays, that you would love to live and work here. Anyway check out the Council's webpage."

Living in the Whitsundays would be like living in my dream, I thought.

I applied and successfully made it through the phone interview. A week later I arrived at Brisbane airport early. I found a seat in the departure lounge within sight of the departure screen. Sitting with book in hand I prepared to destress while waiting to catch my plane to Proserpine. I looked up from my book continuously checking the departure screen. It flashed Proserpine. I looked down at my book listening for the call to board the plane to Proserpine. I didn't hear my call. My heart raced when I rechecked the departure screen. It had changed to Mount Isa. I flew from my chair towards the departure desk. I asked," Did I miss my plane, to Proserpine?"

The Flight Attendant responded, "No Madam. The Proserpine flight has been cancelled. The plane is unsafe to fly. It has been towed for maintenance."

I was taking lots of short shallow breaths, my voice wavered, "But I have a job interview in Proserpine." *They have even taken away my plane,* I thought. For a brief moment I thought that I should run away back home to what I know. It would be easier to stay in the same town, to live in the same house, participate in the same past times and not make major changes.

Now is a good time to run, well it's not my fault that they took away my plane. It's just not meant to be. I could just go home and do what I want, I thought.

"I know I can go home," I mumbled quietly to myself, "but I can't I am already committed to attend an interview in Proserpine. The reason I applied for this job was because I loved the Whitsundays when we visited for a holiday the year before." My dream came true. I got to work in the Whitsundays, live by the sea and walk my dogs on the beach every day. My dream came peppered with challenges.

CHAPTER TWENTY ONE

Developing my awareness even further had spiralled through finding a pea sized lump in my breast. Medical tests proved the lump to be an invasive ductal carcinoma which was apparently as aggressive as it was invasive therefore I was prescribed an aggressive chemotherapy treatment. I had experienced with my son Andrew the devastating effects of chemotherapy and radiotherapy that his doctors chose for him. I was more frightened of the treatment than I was of the consequences, which drove me to find another way to my desired outcome of living a quality life to see my children grow into adulthood and beyond. My journey began with developing awareness around my options to choose the best way forward for me. I explored conventional medicine, mind body healing, homeopathy, and naturopathy for me to choose from this smorgasbord of possibilities. I took the responsibility to focus on the steps of opportunity that I needed to take to reach my outcome of living a quality life to see my children grow up. I needed to use self acuity or self awareness to know what was working, to know what wasn't working and to know what to change and what needed to change. For example I felt fearful to proceed with chemotherapy treatment even though I knew that the cancer that I had removed was aggressive and could return. I knew that I needed to heed my Oncologist's advice and change what I was doing to discourage or prevent cancer from happening to me again. My self awareness around the need to change required that I have the behavioural flexibility to change what doesn't work for me or know how to improve what is working for me.

Having the confidence to make the decisions to make the changes that I needed to in my life to take the best road forward impacted on enriching my whole life in every way. I have met my outcome of preventing the return of cancer that I had removed from my body through taking the responsibility to take make the decisions to take the steps towards meeting my goals whilst focusing on my outcome.

For me the Journey Intensive weekend with Brandon Bays uncovered for me a past experience that I needed to deal with. My son and first born Andrew came up. I remember thinking that my first counsellor was right I hadn't dealt with Andrew's death. Through the Journey intensive processes I learnt to use my imagination to discover how I could choose to identify and deal with major aspects that affected me around the loss of my baby, Andrew. After the first emotional journey process I felt more at peace thinking about Andrew. I continued practicing the processes and found that I had to deal with many different reactions to my issues around Andrew every time he came up in my processes. I have now changed my reaction from feeling sad and guilty around Andrew's passing to responding with gratitude for having the privilege to have had Andrew in my life. In my mind and in my heart I have a strong sense of love and appreciation around Andrew. These processes proved to be so powerful for me. They gave me a tool to peel back the layers of learned emotions which were not always resourceful, like the intensity of pain I felt around losing Andrew that I missed remembering the joy of having Andrew in my life.

I learned how to deal with stuff through awareness, forgiveness and gratitude. Like the time when my back was hurting because I hadn't been walking or exercising. The pain was all too familiar, the thought of which exhausted me. It was Saturday morning and I was home alone.

I sat crossed legged in the quietness of my bedroom where I closed my eyes reaching a deep meditative state. In my mind's eye I climbed down ten steps where I reached an imaginary door. I opened my imaginary door where I met my Mentor. We climbed into my imaginary capsule where we were quickly swept down a beautiful blue clear safe river. We sped towards my destination when I looked across towards my Mentor. He was my true Mentor from many years before. My mentor was a chiropractor,

Peter, who led me to the Silva mind control program that taught me to relax and showed me that I could lead a different life using creative visualisation. In my minds eye my capsule came to a gentle but sudden stop at my backbone which was crooked allowing fluid to drip through my central nervous system in some places and flow rapidly like a waterfall after torrential rains in other areas. As I stood beside the crookedness with my mentor, I could feel heat emanating from the cascading fluid. I felt very warm and suddenly I felt torn. I could see in my mind's eye that I was in the birthing process. I didn't want to leave this safe space and I fought hard not to. I knew the environment out there was hostile. I was being born into an environment that was foreign to my family and my family's culture was different to that around them. I was being pushed out. I gave in to the pressure. I knew that my mum felt sick during my entire incubation never the less she worked hard physically, cleaning, washing, ironing and cooking for many people without the help of technology or electricity.

I imagined that I had hurt my back when I fought the birthing process. Through imaginings I had uncovered my mother's intentions. In my mind's eye or in my imagination my Mother said, "It is scary out there but God will look after you. You just have to believe. Christianity is not about how one behaves or what one believes. Christianity is about forgiveness from God at a soul level. That's when you find true happiness and peace. I have a friend who has it. You can see it shining from her. I want you to have it too. You have to trust in God and live your truth to begin your Journey. It has been my job as your mother to lead you." I realised that my mother, with her strong religious controlling behaviour hadn't hurt me at all. My mum was nurturing me with love and guiding me to a place where she believed I would find peace and happiness.

My mentor had taken me to a safe and protected place where mum and I were immersed in love and protection. This place of safety came through my imagination as I saw that we were on an isolated part of the beach. Through the process I imagined that my younger self was having a conversation with my mum. I realised that she did the best she could with the resources within her. My mum loved her family, even though she didn't often tell us so. Her intentions were influenced through her beliefs and attitudes that were passed down to her through previous generations and through her peers. I understood forgave her, forgave myself for misunderstanding and felt relieved that I had released my old beliefs.

It was so real the tears were pouring down my face, but the experience was amazing like no other that I had ever known. The forgiveness was replaced by an intense feeling of love which surrounded me filling my very soul. This love which has always been there for me is probably the glue that has held my family together through the tapestry of life through which we have grown.

Brandon's Journey Intensive weekend was life changing for me. Those stressful feelings had changed to feelings of a more peaceful nature. The more processes that I did the more at ease I felt. I have discovered that I have no control of 10% of my life, though 90% of my life is decided on how I react. I had reacted with unresourceful or negative thoughts that created negative and unresourceful stressful emotions. Some medical experts say if stress decreases the body's ability to fight disease it loses the ability to kill cancer cells. Other studies have gone as far as to show those women who experienced traumatic life events or losses in previous years had significantly higher rates of breast cancer. I have discovered that I have the resources within me to change how I react to stressful situations. Through using my imagination I can travel along my timeline to access those defining moments that have shaped my life and possibly contributed towards my breast cancer and change my response to them and change my beliefs around them. For example, responding to stressful events with forgiveness and gratitude was a catalyst to lifting stress from me whilst creating a lighter energy that afforded me to experience the sense of peace that is at the core of my being.

I read Brandon's written word and regularly listened to her guided recordings of, '*The Journey*' and '*Freedom Is.*' These learnings that Brandon Bays introduced to me were filtered to become my knowledge, my fears became unfastened, my failures became my successes, I discovered who I am, I learned to be grateful, and I learned to forgive. I felt empowered. Initially I shared process and meditation sessions on a regular basis with a group I met through the Journey Intensive weekend and later continued the processes on my own using the guidance CD's. My journey continues as the more I learn and know the more I realise there is to learn and to know. The rabbit hole is very deep.

Through making choices to move me forward I found the resources within me to deal with the stress. For example I learned to change the stress that came from thinking about the loss of my first son Andrew to appreciating Andrew's gift of sharing his life with him. Andrew taught me so much in such a short time. He showed me his great depth of happiness that was within him, when he looked around and smiled whilst looking at the shiny Christmas decorations. I remember Andrew sitting on the couch beneath the Xmas decorations where he coveted his first Christmas present that he held tightly in his small hand. Andrew smiled broadly as he clutched his teddy bear in one hand, his Duplo truck in the other hand whilst delighting in the shiny Christmas decorations that surrounded him.

I believe that synchronicity led me to attend Brandon Bay's Intensive Journey weekend where I learnt the skills to peel back the layers of emotions to discover my very core to know who I really am. I discovered that awesomeness, that shiny diamond that is at everyone's core.

Through clarity of thought I followed my instincts and found a new specialist in Mackay much closer to home. My Specialist was a caring woman who said, "Two years and six months you have been clear. Did you celebrate at the two year mark?"

"I didn't know that I could. I thought that I had to wait for five years before I got the all clear." I responded.

My Specialist said, "Well given your history and prognosis I would be fairly certain that you are in the clear. I believe that it is unlikely that your breast cancer will return. It is still important that you have your regular mammograms and routine checks as you would anyway. Now go and celebrate."

I had been motivated to take responsibility for my breast cancer journey when chemotherapy treatment was prescribed for me through my fear of my perception around chemotherapy treatment. Chemotherapy treatment seemed incongruent when I chose to believe that there was no cancer left in my body after my mastectomy. I did however need the flexibility to change what I did so that my breast cancer wouldn't return. I used my imagination to use the processes to change my cellular memories so that I could believe that my cellular memories were cleared and that I could live life as if my breast cancer would not return. I chose to believe that when I took responsibility for my breast cancer it was structured around the five success principles.

The first principle of success towards reaching your potential is to know your outcome is to know your desires and set your goals. I chose to model the new thought pattern in the book; *You can heal your life* by Louise Hay, so that I could make a belief around my desired outcome. "It is easy for me to reprogram the computer of my mind. All of life is change, and my mind is ever new."

My outcome focus for my breast cancer journey was to release the stress around the drama of my life to have clarity of mind to choose to change the drama of my life into the adventure of my life: To change the energy that governs my molecules that make my cells which combine to make my organs that make my body work: To clear the negative energy to positive energy within my cells: to change a negative mindset to a positive mindset: to change my body to support the change in my cellular memory to healthy happy cellular memories, to build my resistance around my health through strengthening my mind to strengthen my body to choose my emotions that best serve me and develop my spirituality through self awareness and awareness of what is.

The second success principle is to take the action to achieve your outcome, by taking responsibility for what you focus on. For what you focus on is what you get. I focused on taking small steps towards my bigger goals. I allowed myself to be open to what is and opened my heart to finding the how of what I believed worked for me. I have chosen another new thought pattern from *"You can heal your life,"* by Louise Hay. *"I lovingly forgive and release all of the past. I choose to fill my world with joy. I love and approve of myself."* That served me through my breast cancer journey. I used the processes for change that I learnt from Brandon Bay's

Intensive weekend workshop that I subsequently practiced through her recorded guided meditation CD's.

The third success principle is to use self acuity to have awareness around the congruency of your actions to ensure that they are taking you towards your outcome. When choosing to do meditation and journey work for my breast cancer healing journey I would refer back to what I had learnt in the Silva mind control seminar some fifteen years earlier, to check that I could trust my belief that I was on the right path. I noticed that as my journey progressed I was beginning to feel happier. I adopted another one of Louise Hay's new thought patterns to make a belief that *"I am important. I do count. I now nourish myself with love and with joy. I allow others the freedom to be who they are. We are all safe and free."*

The fourth success principle is about having the behavioural flexibility to change what doesn't serve you to achieve your outcome to what is resourceful to get the results that you want. I did that earlier on in my journey where I chose not to go with the prescribed chemotherapy treatment. When I thought about me having chemotherapy my mind filled with distressing thoughts and I felt unease. I was open to listen to what was on offer and what could be. I weighed up my options that were presented to me around probability based on statistics. I knew I had to do something differently or the same may happen again. I chose to trust my feelings and my inner knowing that I would choose the best way forward for me.

The fifth principle is about creating within you a psychology and physiology of excellence to create the result you want. To quote Louise Hay, *"only by practicing over and over do we learn the new and make it a natural part of us."* I learned and practiced what I had learned and learned some more. I felt better and better every day. People told me how much better I looked every day. Psychiatrist RD Laing says, "Change your body change your mind, change your mind change your body."

Reminiscing I realise that my cancer journey opened the magic door of discovery for me. I discovered through my imagination in my mind's eye the door to my soul. I found that the energy that governs the molecules that make the cells combine to make the organs that make me work. I discovered that this energy that is so powerful expands my being to more than just my human form. Who we really are is an energy of pure potential made up of love, light and limitless possibility and what prevents us from tapping into our real selves is negative emotions fear and self imposed limitations. Learning how to overcome fear and self imposed limitations led me to access the feelings of love, joy, gratitude and forgiveness that have empowered my very being. My road to discovery culminated with finding a small lump the size of a pea that signalled me to face my greatest fear that turned me towards my journey of self discovery. I have learned through my Neuro Linguistic Programming (NLP) training with Robb Whitewood that our journey in life is about travelling from the present to the future passing goal posts on the way. The vehicle we use to get there is the methodology of travel for our journey. "The vehicle is frequently inherited from family, friends, cultures, socio-economics or religion. Some people choose to walk, others run, and others just drive. It can be of course be traded in at any time you choose." Through using our imagination we can discover our defining moments and go back in time to change how we reacted to those moments. We can change our thoughts, our feelings and our beliefs to change our vehicle and our state to enjoy the journey of adventure that is called life. I learned to make changes at an unconscious level for change at a conscious level. I trusted my subconscious to lead me to the appropriate change methodology that I needed at the time. I believe that through using my imagination I have entered the rabbit hole, to deepen my self awareness experience to feel better, to be better and better every day in every way.

Albert Einstein says, "Imagination is more important than knowledge. For knowledge is limited to all we now know and understand while imagination embraces the entire world and all there ever will be to know and understand."

I had used my imagination to take me from my greatest fear of having breast cancer happen to me towards my greatest discovery that I could take the responsibility for how I reacted to my life's happenings where I discovered my greatest success that through using my imagination I could change my mind to change my body to feel better and better every day.

ACKNOWLEDGEMENTS

I acknowledge Brandon Bay's significant contribution to my cancer journey through her spoken and written word and my attendance at her intensive journey seminar.

I acknowledge Ian Gawler, Shivani Goodman, Hose Siva, and Louise Hays for inspiring me through my attendance at their seminars or reading their written words.

I also acknowledge the medical people, the doctors and the nurses who took care of me and the alternative practitioners who took the time with me to learn how they could best help me.

I would like to thank my family and friends for their support.

I acknowledge my friend Natasha Jochim who inspired me to write and I am grateful for her belief in me.

www.ingramcontent.com/pod-product-compliance
Lightning Source LLC
Chambersburg PA
CBHW020421290526
45785CB00002B/672